PASS USMLE Step 1

PASS USMLE Step 1: Practice by Assessing Study Skills

Judy A. Schwenker, M.S.
Coordinator, Student Academic Support,
Medical College of Wisconsin, Milwaukee

Little, Brown and Company
Boston New York Toronto London

First Edition

Library of Congress Cataloging-in-Publication Data

Schwenker, Judy A.
PASS USMLE Step 1: practice by assessing study skills / Judy A. Schwenker.
p. cm.
Includes bibliographical references and index.
ISBN 0-316-77600-9
1. Medicine—Examinations, questions, etc. 2. Medical sciences—Examinations, questions, etc. I. Title.
[DNLM: 1. Medicine—examinations questions. W 18 S4139p 1995]
R834.5.S39 1995
610'.76—dc20
DNLM/DLC
for Library of Congress 94-45448
CIP

Printed in the United States of America

Fig. 3-6 reprinted from Bullock J (ed): Physiology. Baltimore: Williams & Wilkins, 1984.

Editorial: Evan R. Schnittman
Production Editor: Anne Holm
Copyeditor: Libby Dabrowski
Indexer: Mary Duffy
Production Supervisor: Cate Rickard
Cover Designer: Cate Rickard

Contents

Contributing Authors

Nabil J. Alkayed, M.D.
Professor of Physiology, Medical College of Wisconsin, Milwaukee

Rebekha Grabher-Neu, M.D.
Resident, PG IV, Department of Pathology, Medical College of Wisconsin; Resident, PG IV, Department of Pathology, Doyne Hospital, Milwaukee

Thomas C. Herzig, Ph.D.
Postdoctoral Fellow, Department of Physiology, Medical College of Wisconsin, Milwaukee

J. Kevin Langford, M.S.
Graduate Student/Research Assistant, Department of Cellular Biology and Anatomy, Medical College of Wisconsin, Milwaukee

Kevin P. Raisch, Ph.D.
Research Scientist, Department of Microbiology, Medical College of Wisconsin, Milwaukee

David L. Roberts, Ph.D.
Postdoctoral Fellow, Department of Biochemistry, Medical College of Wisconsin, Milwaukee

Jacqueline R. Roberts, Ph.D.
Postdoctoral Fellow, Department of Biochemistry, Medical College of Wisconsin, Milwaukee

Blair E. Taylor, Ph.D.
Postdoctoral Research Associate, Endocrinology-Reproductive Physiology Program, University of Wisconsin-Madison, Madison, Wisconsin

Preface

PASS USMLE Step 1: Practice by Assessing Study Skills is the product of 14 years of working with medical students from the time of orientation to medical school through commencement. During those years, students have been both my joy and my inspiration. In helping them to cope with the pace and volume demands of the basic science courses and to prepare for the licensure examinations, I have been challenged as well. My challenge has been to understand what keeps students from performing well on examinations, especially on large standardized (multiple-choice) examinations, and then to draw on my background in learning theory to develop solutions to the students' problems. This book summarizes what my students have taught me about test-taking problems and what we discovered together as we worked to help them become better test takers. While I felt no small degree of trepidation in agreeing to try to develop these insights into book form, many students encouraged me by volunteering to read the draft and provide feedback. I am deeply grateful for their kindness and their input.

This book is intended to be used over a period of months as you begin preparing to take Step 1, the first of three parts of the USMLE. In it you will find practical approaches to choosing review materials, which are often helpful while you are taking a course. There is also a lengthy chapter on strategies for improving how you read, interpret, and reason through answer choices on multiple-choice test items. For that chapter alone, it may be worth spending time with the book during your first year in medical school, rather than during the final month or so before you take Step 1. As with any skill, practice is important, and you will have ample opportunities to try test strategies during the basic science courses.

The final chapter contains practice questions arranged by subject so that it will be easier to use during your review. These items are representative of what you will see on Step 1 and will provide you with the chance to try the strategies that are introduced in Chapter 2. I think you will find that different sections of the book are helpful at different stages in the process of preparing for Step 1. I sincerely hope you will find it readable and useful and that it will serve as an antidote to the anxiety that is so common among second-year medical students as the examination date approaches. By following a rational, analytical approach to preparing for the examination, you can be confident of doing your best both in reviewing for Step 1 and in taking it. The best of luck on your "road to Boards."

J. A. S.

Acknowledgments

This book would never have been written but for the significant help and encouragement I received from many people. I want to thank my husband, Erich, who believed that I had something important to say, and also my children, who put up with a distracted parent who spent so many hours in front of the word processor. I want to acknowledge the special assistance of two colleagues, Patricia Sorcic and Betty Strecker, who gave of their computer talents and kindness in equal measure. Thanks also go to my medical colleagues who reviewed test items and developed explanations for test items: J. Kevin Langford, M.S.; Kevin P. Raisch, Ph.D.; Jacqueline R. Roberts, Ph.D.; David L. Roberts, Ph.D.; Nabil J. Alkayed, M.D.; Thomas C. Herzig, Ph.D.; Blair E. Taylor, Ph.D.; and Rebekha Grabher-Neu, M.D. I also deeply appreciate the guidance and support I received from Evan R. Schnittman, medical editor at Little, Brown and Company, who suggested that I write this book and was so helpful throughout the process, and George Weymer, medical sales representative at Little, Brown, who believed that students would benefit and first proposed the idea to my publisher. Finally, I want to express my appreciation to the students at the Medical College of Wisconsin. By seeking my help and sharing their difficulties and joys over the past 14 years, they gave me the opportunity to reflect, invent, teach, and better understand the process of learning medical information. They were my mentors as much as I was theirs.

Introduction

There are many review materials for the USMLE Step 1: There are book series that summarize each of the basic science subjects and others that offer hundreds of practice questions with content explanations for each item on all subject areas assessed in Step 1. *PASS USMLE Step 1: Practice by Assessing Study Skills* is different. While it contains hundreds of practice items, its basic purpose is to guide you through the process of reviewing and to teach you how to become a better test taker on multiple-choice examinations of all kinds. This book will help you design a review plan and study schedule based on your unique profile of strengths and weaknesses in basic science subjects and on the amount of time you have available for reviewing for Step 1. You will learn criteria that you can use to select review materials systematically, rather than basing your decisions on the advice of other students whose learning styles and academic profiles may be very different from your own. This book, then, aims to teach you a **process** by which you can prepare in order to succeed on Step 1 and on many other examinations in the future.

Chapter 1 is a practice test that you should take before beginning to design a review plan. Chapter 2 discusses many of the practice questions from Chapter 1 to illustrate test-taking techniques. Each strategy is demonstrated in the context of an actual question, so that you will know when to use it.

Error analysis, a method of looking systematically at your errors, is explained. You will then be able to use it to sort the errors you made on the initial practice test into meaningful categories. And you will be able to make decisions about what you need to review based on empirical data on your performance rather than on guesses as to what you think your strengths and weaknesses are. It helps you become aware of the types of errors you are prone to making, so that you can take steps to avoid making similar errors in the future.

Chapter 2 is designed to help you become test savvy before you sit for Step 1. Test questions are analyzed, and reasoning strategies are modeled with test items like those you will find on Step 1. You will become adept at using sophisticated, reasoned approaches to questions, and this will allow you to be a far more confident and successful test taker.

My work with students over many years has shown that medical students, being bright and successful students as undergraduates, have rarely been taught sophisticated test-taking techniques. After all, if you are already achieving scores higher than those of most of your classmates in college, why should you need any instruction in how to approach test items or how to make better educated guesses? Yet you are now competing against a national population of medical students who are much like you. Some have stumbled across strategic test-taking techniques and have used them with great success throughout the first 2 years of medical school. These students are often mentioned by classmates as the ones who do better on tests than others even when they don't appear to know the material any more thoroughly than their peers.

Students who have not learned how to approach multiple-choice examinations strategically are at an increasing disadvantage when they have to compete to "show what they know" on standardized, objective examinations. They often feel, and rightfully so, that they know much more than their scores indicate. If you are this type of student, make the effort to work through this book. Standardized tests don't disappear after Step 1. From clinical rotation final examinations to specialty boards, you will need to deal with multiple-choice tests for many years to come, so it is worth the investment of time and effort to become a better test taker right now.

This book offers systematic approaches to items on multiple-choice examinations that will improve your chances of achieving as high a score as possible with the level of learned information you bring into the Step 1 examination room. If you work through the book carefully and make a genuine attempt to apply what you have learned as you take Step 1, you will make fewer errors, make a higher percentage of correct educated guesses, and feel more confident and less anxious. The strategies in this book will work with any type of multiple-choice test. They work in conjunction with recalled information. They are not gimmicks.

Effective test strategies allow you to draw on both sides of your brain. They encourage you to use reason to complement your knowledge base as you think through questions and help you broaden your perspective on items. You will learn to use more than just the facts you scrambled to cram into your brain during a few weeks of frantic reviewing in order to answer questions.

Because you need to gain a sense of when and how each strategy is used, all test strategies are taught in relation to actual questions. This part of the book will read somewhat like a dialogue taking place between you and an expert test taker. First, a question will be presented and you will be asked to answer the question. Then, while your own reasoning is fresh in your mind, you will be shown the thought process that an expert test taker used in thinking through that same item. By comparing your own approach to the expert's, you will come to appreciate how each strategy works, what type of item it works with, and how strategies work in synergistic ways with a test taker's knowledge base.

A second practice test is provided in Chapter 3. This will give you the opportunity to apply the strategies that you have learned and to determine the progress you have made by becoming more test-wise. Again, certain items are analyzed following each section of the second practice test to demonstrate the strategies applicable to each item, in order to reinforce what you have learned.

Description of the USMLE Step 1

The USMLE Step 1 is a 2-day examination containing approximately 800 items. It is administered in four booklets, two each day, with 3 hours allowed for each booklet. The items are presented in standard multiple-choice formats. The formats are grouped within each booklet, with standard directions presented at the head of each format grouping. A table of normal laboratory values is also included in each booklet. **There is no content organization within the examination.** This means that a biochemistry item can be followed by a cell biology item, a pathology item, an embryology item, and so on. This aspect is unique to Step 1 and is unfamiliar to most medical students because most medical school tests assess a single content area at a time. This is one reason why it is recommended that students preparing for Step 1 take at least one practice test that simulates the item mixing of Step 1. The constant switching of frame of reference from one item to the next takes some getting used to. Accordingly, the first practice test in this book is in item-scrambled format.

Two item formats are used in Step 1. Single best answer (SBA) items, both positively and negatively phrased, which are the most frequently used type of question on multiple-choice examinations. These consist of a statement, or question stem, followed by a list of three to five options. In Step 1, the options are always lettered (A, B, C, D, E). Incorrect options can be partially correct, with the test taker instructed to pick the best of the lettered options for each item.

The negatively phrased SBA items are signaled by a boldface word such as **least, not**, or **except**. While most students are familiar with this type of item, on a long examination, fatigue can lead to a higher percentage of errors on negatively phrased items because the test taker working through a long, wordy stem and list of options may forget that he or she is looking for the one that is **not** correct and accept the next true option, resulting in an erroneous answer to the item.

The second item format used in Step 1 is the matching format. Such items are arranged in clusters that relate to a single topic. This allows the items to share a single list of response options, which can range in length from 4 to 26 options. The options are usually listed alphabetically. Again, several options may be partially correct, but the test taker is directed to select the best option from the list. Each option can be used once, more than once, or not at all. There are specific strategies to use with these matching items to avoid spending too much time on them. These will be discussed later. The significant point is that not many medical students are used to the longer matching sets that contain up to 26 options, because few medical schools have scoring programs that can accommodate this many responses to an item on a computer-scored answer sheet. For this reason, it is advisable for students to seek out practice items in this format to become comfortable with longer lists of options and to practice answering them in an efficient manner.

The USMLE is constructed according to an integrated content outline that assesses basic science material along three dimensions: (1) organizational level, (2) process, and (3) system. Within each dimension, items are apportioned to subcategories of normal and abnormal and to levels such as organ, tissue, or single-cell. The items have been designed to assess not only your knowledge but also your judgment in evaluation, reasoning, and discrimination. Areas such as these frequently cross the line between one basic science subject area and another. Descriptions of laboratory situations or problem scenarios in the clinical setting are frequent lead-ins to items.

Step 1 is scored and reported on three-digit and two-digit scales. A three-digit passing score is 176, while a score of 75 is a passing score on the two-digit scale. The three-digit score is a standardized score with a defined mean of 200 and a standard deviation of 20 points. The passing rate is normally about 90% for medical students taking the examination for the first time at the end of the second year of medical school.

There is no particular advantage derived by taking Step 1 in September rather than June, because the procedures used by the National Board of Medical Examiners provide examinees with a consistent standard from one test administration to the next. Thus your decision as to when to take Step 1 should be based on a consideration of which time frame allows for the degree of personal energy and review time you want to bring to the preparation process. You should also investigate any resources that your medical school may make available to students preparing for Step 1. Some schools make passing Step 1 a condition of academic advancement, so you should investigate your school's policy before registering for Step 1.

PASS USMLE Step 1

1

How to Use the Diagnostic Pretest

In order to get the most out of the time you spend preparing for Step 1, you need to take some time before your review process begins to reflect on your own test-taking behaviors. If you have acquired some bad habits or failed to acquire some test-taking strategies, rushing out to buy the bestselling review book for each subject won't cure the problem. This is why students who feel prepared for exams aren't always happy with the results.

Take an hour or two now to work through the Diagnostic Pretest. Chapter 2 draws on many items in the Pretest for examples of strategies, and therefore it will be helpful to have worked through the items yourself first. In addition, you will need this "raw data" on your test-taking habits to learn how to analyze your own test behavior based on how you answered the Pretest items. A scoring key is provided following the Pretest for you to use in evaluating your responses. The items are mixed together, not grouped by subject, to give you a taste of what Step 1 is like.

Don't feel as though you need to study before taking the Pretest. Subsequent sections will guide you through an analysis of your performance and discuss what implications various error patterns have for reviewing and practicing for Step 1.

1. A 32-year-old office worker, complaining of shortness of breath, had pulmonary function testing that resulted in a diagnosis of pulmonary fibrosis. Which of the sets of values below is consistent with this diagnosis?
   A. $FEV_1/FVC = 82\%$, IC = 3.4 L, FRC = 2.80 L, and TV = 500 ml
   B. FVC = 3.20 L, FEV_1 = 2.00 L, TLC = 6.20 L, and RV = 3.00 L
   C. $FEV_1/FVC = 54\%$, FRC = 4.80 L, and RV = 2.30 L
   D. FVC = 2.00 L, FEV_1 = 1.80 L, TLC = 3.00 L, and RV = 1.00 L
   E. None of these value sets is consistent with the diagnosis.

2. Which of the following serves as a precursor for testosterone?
   A. estrone
   B. cholesterol
   C. aldosterone
   D. cortisol
   E. estriol

3. Conduction velocity along a myelinated nerve fiber is
   A. directly proportional to fiber diameter
   B. directly proportional to extracellular resistance

C. inversely proportional to the thickness of the myelin coat
D. directly proportional to the extent of demyelination
E. inversely proportional to temperature

4. Which of the following sequences of enzyme activities is required for excision/repair of DNA?
A. endonuclease, exonuclease, polymerase, ligase
B. exonuclease, endonuclease, polymerase, ligase
C. exonuclease, polymerase, endonuclease, ligase
D. polymerase, exonuclease, endonuclease, ligase
E. exonuclease, ligase, polymerase, endonuclease

5. The length of hospitalization for eight patients who underwent a new procedure for the treatment of acute gout exacerbations was 10, 8, 7, 7, 4, 9, 9, and 6 days. The mean length of stay for this group of patients is
A. 8.1 days
B. 7.8 days
C. 7.2 days
D. 7.5 days
E. 7.1 days

6. The range of stay for the eight patients described above is
A. 4 days
B. 5.5 days
C. 6 days
D. 7 days
E. 7.5 days

7. Which of the following cells removes immune complexes from the bloodstream?
A. B cells
B. basophils
C. Kupffer cells
D. plasma cells
E. T cells

8. An uncoupler of oxidative phosphorylation causes
A. an increase in electron transport and an increase in ATP synthesis
B. a decrease in electron transport and a decrease in ATP synthesis
C. a decrease in electron transport and an increase in ATP synthesis
D. an increase in electron transport and a decrease in ATP synthesis
E. a decrease in heat production during electron transport

9. Which of the following has the **lowest** metabolic clearance rate?
A. hormone A with a half-life of 1 hour, 95% plasma binding
B. hormone B with a half-life of 1 minute, 5% plasma binding
C. hormone C with a half-life of 1 hour, 60% of plasma binding
D. hormone D with a half-life of 1 day, 99% plasma binding
E. hormone E with a half-life of 1 minute, 0.5% plasma binding

10. In performing a venous cutdown for IV access, the most commonly used site is
    A. at the anterior tibial muscle origin
    B. just lateral to the Achilles tendon
    C. anterior to the medial malleolus
    D. in the popliteal fossa
    E. between the fourth and fifth metatarsals on the dorsum of the foot

11. If half of a drug is in the nonionized form at a pH of 5.0, what is the pKa of the drug?
    A. 3
    B. 4
    C. 5
    D. 6
    E. 7

12. Damage to which of the following nerves might lead to an inability to abduct the arm?
    A. median
    B. posterior interosseus
    C. musculocutaneous
    D. lateral pectoral
    E. axillary

13. Which of the following statements regarding child abuse **is not** true?
    A. Mothers are less likely than fathers to abuse their children.
    B. Normal term children are less likely to be abused than are premature ones.
    C. Older children are less likely to be abused than are children under the age of three.
    D. Many abusing parents were themselves abused as children.
    E. Frequently, one child in a family is singled out for abuse.

14. The liver synthesizes all of the following entities **except**
    A. chylomicrons
    B. low-density lipoproteins
    C. ketone bodies
    D. high-density lipoproteins
    E. bile acid

15. Which of the following amino acids has a side chain functional group with the most alkaline pH?
    A. cysteine
    B. leucine
    C. lysine
    D. histidine
    E. aspartate

16. Abdominal masses in newborns are most commonly due to which of the following conditions?
    A. hepatomegaly
    B. hydronephrosis

C. mesenteric cysts
D. ovarian tumors
E. splenomegaly

Items 17–21

Match the one choice from the list of urinary stone substances that is most closely associated with each question. Each choice may be used once, more than once, or not at all.

A. calcium oxalate
B. calcium phosphate
C. magnesium ammonium phosphate
D. uric acid
E. cystine

17. Formed in infected alkaline urine.
18. Most common form of stone in the United States.
19. Radiolucent stones in patients with gout.
20. Associated with hyperparathyroidism.
21. Occurs in children with an inborn error of metabolism.

22. A 35-year-old female patient's eyes move normally except that her left eye cannot adduct. You suspect that her CNS lesion involves the
    A. IV nucleus on the left side
    B. VI nucleus on the right side
    C. medulla
    D. left medial longitudinal fasciculus
    E. right cerebellum

23. Urea is the product of a reaction catalyzed by
    A. an aminotransferase requiring pyridoxal phosphate
    B. a complex of enzymes requiring derivatives of riboflavin, thiamine, and pantothenic acid
    C. the hydrolase, glutaminase
    D. a complex of enzymes requiring aspartic acid, *N*-acetyl glutamic acid, and ascorbic acid
    E. the hydrolase, arginase

24. Which of the following **is not** a normal stage in the grieving process following the death of a close family member?
    A. Turning to others to fill the emotional void left by the death.
    B. Keeping one's feelings about the deceased private.
    C. Realizing the depth of affection felt toward the deceased.
    D. Wanting to talk about negative feelings associated with the deceased.
    E. A firm realization and acceptance of the person's death.

Items 25–27

Select the appropriate mechanism of action for each of the antibiotics listed below.

A. Inhibits synthesis of steroids.
B. Inhibits cell wall synthesis.
C. Reversibly binds to 50 S ribosome subunits.
D. Inhibits aminoacyl RNA binding to 50 S subunits.
E. Binds to 30 S ribosome subunits.

25. streptomycin
26. penicillin G
27. chloramphenicol

Items 28–32

Match the one choice from the list that is most commonly associated with each question. Each choice may be used once, more than once, or not at all.

A. primary hyperparathyroidism
B. secondary hyperparathyroidism
C. resistance to PTH action (defective PTH receptors)
D. vitamin D intoxication
E. total parathyroidectomy

28. patient with hypercalcemia, hyperphosphatemia, low PTH
29. patient with hypocalcemia, hyperphosphatemia, low PTH
30. patient with hypocalcemia, hypophosphatemia, high PTH
31. patient with hypercalcemia, hypophosphatemia, high PTH
32. patient with hypocalcemia, hyperphosphatemia, high PTH

33. The principal function of myocardial ATP is in
   A. protein synthesis
   B. the uptake of calcium by the sarcoplasmic reticulum
   C. the formation of cyclic AMP
   D. contractile activity
   E. generating reduced oxygen species

34. Which of the following values is always **less than** alveolar pressure in a normal person?
   A. pressure inside the trachea
   B. pulmonary capillary pressure
   C. pleural pressure
   D. transpulmonary pressure
   E. pressure inside the bronchioles

35. The cerebrospinal fluid is formed primarily by
   A. blood capillary cells throughout the brain parenchyma
   B. endothelial cells in blood capillaries of the choroid plexus
   C. epithelial cells of the arachnoid granulations
   D. epithelial cells of the choroid plexus
   E. ependymal cells lining the ventricles

36. Old age onset of fragile skin, loss of suppleness, and a high degree of wrinkling is common in patients with
   A. Addison's disease
   B. cutis laxa

C. Ehlers-Danlos syndrome
D. hereditary albinism, old age–onset type
E. overexposure to the sun

37. Which vitamin plays a key role in the prevention of lactic acid production during ethanol metabolism?
A. thiamine
B. vitamin A
C. vitamin C
D. vitamin B_{12}
E. cholecalciferol

38. Four weeks ago, a 24-year-old woman had a hydatidiform mole evacuated. Now she shows increased levels of human chorionic gonadotropin in her peripheral blood. All of the following might be reasonable **except** that she
A. may have an invasive mole
B. may have a choriocarcinoma
C. should be given chemotherapy
D. should be put on oral contraceptives
E. All of these are reasonable.

39. All of the following factors can contribute to patient noncompliance with prescribed medications **except**
A. the physician fails to explain the reason for the prescription
B. the patient is elderly and lives alone
C. the prescription regimen requires once-a-day dosing
D. the symptoms lessen
E. side effects occur

40. The brain area most involved in controlling hunger is the
A. amygdala
B. cerebellum
C. substantia nigra
D. hypothalamus
E. hippocampus

41. Which of the following signs suggests a diagnosis of primary aldosteronism?
A. increased circulating catecholamines
B. increased circulating renin
C. pressure gradient between upper and lower parts of the body
D. low plasma potassium
E. marked elevation in plasma creatinine concentration

Items 42–45

Match each instance of behavior with its appropriate defense mechanism. The choices may be used once, more than once, or not at all.

A. introjection
B. projection

C. sublimation
D. reaction formation
E. denial

42. A 35-year-old woman is told that she has terminal liver cancer. A week later, she claims that her doctors cannot determine what is wrong with her.
43. An elderly, intellectually alert man is extremely upset about being placed in a nursing home and insists that the staff hate him and verbally abuse him.
44. A young man, not athletically talented but with many close friends on college teams, decides to open a sports equipment and memorabilia store next door to the college sports arena.
45. A young, married professional woman who resents having to work and fears her boss repeatedly tells her friends and family how much she loves being a liberated professional person.

46. Antibodies are used in both research and clinical applications. Which of the following procedures **does not** directly use antibodies?
A. Western blot
B. radioimmunoassay
C. catalytic antibodies
D. immunofluorescence
E. Southern blot

47. Which of the following hormones would you associate with nonvascular cell contraction?
A. antidiuretic hormone
B. luteinizing hormone
C. oxytocin
D. prolactin
E. thyroid-stimulating hormone

48. You are treating a 67-year-old diabetic man who takes insulin. You wish to prescribe medication to control his recently diagnosed hypertension. Which of the following drugs should be given with caution and only with careful education of this patient?
A. alpha methyldopa (Aldomet)
B. guanethidine (Ismelin)
C. hydralazine
D. prazosin (Minipress)
E. propranolol (Inderal)

49. Ovarian cells that transform into the corpus luteum must have receptors for
A. epidermal growth factor
B. follicle-stimulating hormone
C. inhibin
D. luteinizing hormone
E. progesterone

50. A patient who has suffered an inversion injury to the ankle joint presents with pain and swelling over the lateral malleolus area. Which of the following ligaments is most likely to have been damaged?
   A. long plantar
   B. anterior talofibular ligament
   C. deltoid ligament
   D. spring ligament
   E. None of these is likely to have been damaged.

51. Two different enzymes are isolated from widely divergent organisms and found to catalyze the same biochemical reactions. Which property would the two enzymes have in common?
   A. the V^{max} for their reactions
   B. the equilibrium constant for their reactions
   C. their protein molecular weights
   D. the K^{m} for substrate binding
   E. the energy of activation for their reactions

52. Pseudostratified ciliated epithelium is found in all of the following sites **except** the
   A. alveolar duct
   B. bronchiole
   C. bronchus
   D. larynx
   E. nasopharynx

53. All of the following typify IgA nephropathy (Berger's disease) **except**
   A. it may result from injury of the intestinal mucosa by lectin-like molecules from wheat
   B. it may be associated with alcohol abuse
   C. deposits of IgA, IgG, and C3 are found in the mesangium
   D. it frequently progresses to end-stage renal disease
   E. its course is generally considered to be benign

54. Which of the following compounds is a carrier of the hydroxyethyl derivative formed during the conversion of pyruvate to acetyl-CoA?
   A. antothenic acid
   B. biotin
   C. nicotinamide
   D. carnitine
   E. thiamine pyrophosphate

55. The migrating motor complex in the small intestine is absent after
   A. bilateral thoracic truncal vagotomy
   B. superior and inferior ganglionectomy
   C. IV bolus injection of motilin
   D. ingestion of a meal
   E. None of the above is correct.

56. Disulfiram (Antabuse) programs treat chronic alcoholism by explicitly employing which of the following techniques?

A. implosive therapy
B. counterconditioning
C. cognitive therapy
D. systematic desensitization
E. aversive deconditioning

57. Which of the following disorders could be called a REM pattern disorder?
A. hypnagogia
B. insomnia
C. somnambulism
D. narcolepsy
E. night terrors

58. The most common etiology of primary hyperparathyroidism is
A. osteomalacia
B. parathyroid adenoma
C. parathyroid carcinoma
D. primary parathyroid gland hyperplasia
E. renal failure

59. Which of the following studies is most helpful in the diagnosis of congenital adrenal hyperplasia?
A. buccal smear
B. exploratory laparotomy
C. genitogram
D. karyotype
E. urinary 17-ketosteroids

60. The pressure-volume loop of the left ventricle is most likely to be displaced upward and to the right and to exhibit an increase in the loop area in response to
A. mitral stenosis
B. mitral regurgitation
C. pulmonic stenosis
D. intraventricular septal defect with left-to-right shunt
E. aortic stenosis

61. By definition, a carcinoma is described by all of the following **except**
A. epithelial in origin
B. gland-forming
C. malignant
D. neoplastic
E. a subtype of cancer

62. Which of the following factors most strongly affects the social development of a child?
A. the degree of permissiveness of the parents
B. the parents' love for each other
C. the type of punishment used
D. the birth order
E. the emotional climate created by the parents

63. Blood glucose can derive from all of the following **except**
    A. alanine from dietary peptides
    B. degradation of liver glycogen
    C. lactose from milk
    D. protein breakdown in hepatectomized animals
    E. glycerol from dietary fats

64. All of the following can occur during the processing of mammalian mRNA **except**
    A. cleavage of a 5' leader sequence
    B. clapping of the 5' end
    C. removal of intervening sequences
    D. ligation of exons
    E. polyadenylation of the 3' end

65. When alcohol use among women and men was examined, each of the following was found to be true **except**
    A. there is a greater societal tolerance for heavy drinking in men
    B. women drink less in mixed company
    C. alcoholic women as a group incur greater societal costs than do male alcoholics as a group
    D. there are fewer female than male alcoholics
    E. male and female alcoholics suffer comparable rates of morbidity and mortality

66. Which of the following is a correct statement about glycogen?
    A. It contains close to equal numbers of alpha-1,4 and alpha-1,6 linkages.
    B. It is absent in most patients with glycogen storage disease.
    C. The number of reducing ends equals the number of nonreducing ends.
    D. It is the major source of energy in the resting human body.
    E. It is stored in the cytoplasm of liver cells.

67. In a patient with hyperammonemia, exhibiting low citrulline and low orotate, the enzyme most likely to be deficient is
    A. arginase
    B. carbamyl phosphate synthetase
    C. arginosuccinase
    D. arginosuccinic acid synthetase
    E. ornithine transcarbamylase

68. Identify the characteristic of a laboratory test that **is least** important to consider before ordering.
    A. the specificity of the test
    B. the likelihood of a significant result
    C. the sensitivity of the test
    D. the degree of pain and discomfort of the test for the patient
    E. the availability of the test on the clinic premises

69. Which of the following systems appears to be most sensitive to prenatal viral infection in the fetus?

A. cardiovascular
B. digestive
C. musculoskeletal
D. nervous
E. respiratory

70. A 47-year-old accountant presents with a chief complaint of stomach pain for the last week. In what order should you proceed with the abdominal examination?
A. inspection-auscultation-palpation-percussion
B. inspection-palpation-auscultation-percussion
C. inspection-palpation-percussion-auscultation
D. palpation-auscultation-inspection-percussion
E. inspection-percussion-auscultation-palpation

71. Long-term regulation of arterial blood pressure
A. is independent of carotid sinus reflexes
B. is affected by the renin-angiotensin system
C. depends on renal excretory function
D. is markedly affected by changes in salt and water balance
E. is regulated by all of the above factors

72. Regeneration properties of peripheral and central neurons differ in
A. the changes in their ultrastructure during chromatolysis
B. their ability to form initial sprouts after axotomy
C. their ability to significantly elongate an axon after injury
D. their vulnerability to physical injury
E. their ability to replace dead neurons by proliferation

73. In the normal adult, needle puncture of the spinal dura and arachnoid matter in order to withdraw CSF should be made caudal to
A. T12
B. L1
C. L2
D. S2
E. S5

74. During which stage of the life cycle are depression and suicide most common?
A. early adolescence (11–15 years)
B. old age (>65 years)
C. middle age (35–65 years)
D. late adolescence (16–21 years)
E. early adulthood (21–35 years)

75. Classic herniation (the most common type) of the intervertebral disk between vertebrae would put pressure on which of the following spinal nerves?
A. L2
B. L3
C. L4

D. L5
E. S1

76. Which of the following acts by selectively inhibiting monoamine oxidase F and is used to treat parkinsonism?
A. carbidopa
B. phenelzine
C. deprenyl
D. bromocriptine
E. tranylcypromine

77. A parent who has lost an infant to illness decides to return to college to train as an elementary school teacher. This behavior is called
A. denial
B. reaction formation
C. reversal
D. displacement
E. depression

78. Subacute endocarditis is associated with all of the following **except**
A. rheumatically damaged heart valves
B. IV drug abuse
C. organisms of low pathogenicity such as alpha-hemolytic streptococci
D. congenitally abnormal hearts
E. positive blood cultures

79. Which of the following disorders **does not** mimic Alzheimer-type dementia in the elderly patient?
A. coronary artery disease
B. cancer
C. medication side effects and interactions
D. depression
E. stroke

80. By definition, a pathologic fracture means that the involved bone
A. has formed a callus
B. is healing with a pseudoarthrosis
C. is infected
D. is malignant
E. was abnormal before it broke

Items 81–84

Match each drug to its potential side effects.

A. depression
B. impaired concentration, drowsiness
C. dyskinesia
D. acute psychotic states
E. mood elevation

81. propranolol
82. scopolamine
83. L–dopa
84. nicotine withdrawal

85. A patient presents with fullness in the outer quadrant of the left breast and a slight change in texture over this region for the past 2 months. The physical examination reveals a slight tenderness but no palpable abnormality. She is 42 and previously in good health. Your first step should be to
    A. obtain serum estrogen and progesterone levels
    B. order a mammogram
    C. perform a fine needle aspiration of the area
    D. perform an excisional biopsy of the area
    E. reassure her and have her return in 2 months

86. Which of the following best defines the concept of relative risk (RR)?
    A. The probability that a person who is exposed to a certain disease will, in fact, contract the disease.
    B. The incidence of a disease.
    C. The probability that someone who has a certain disease has been exposed to a particular risk factor for that disease.
    D. The ratio of the incidence of a disease among risk-exposed individuals to the incidence among nonrisk-exposed individuals.
    E. The excess of disease that can be attributed to a particular risk factor for that disease.

87. Which of the following conditions would most likely require a pacemaker?
    A. sinus bradycardia
    B. atrial flutter
    C. third-degree heart block
    D. ventricular tachycardia
    E. sinus arrhythmia

88. All of the following are used to treat asthma **except**
    A. corticosteroids
    B. theophylline
    C. cromolyn sodium
    D. dextromethorphan
    E. beta-adrenergic agonists

89. Which of the following **does not** generally contribute to reduced airway flow rates as measured by spirometry?
    A. hypertrophy of airway smooth muscle
    B. mucosal or submucosal swelling of airways
    C. increased airway secretions
    D. bronchospasm
    E. increased alveolar connection tissue

90. A 59-year-old postmenopausal woman presents with a pruritic, whitish vulvar lesion of 1 month's duration. Your first step should be to

A. prescribe a topical antipruritic medication
B. schedule her for laser surgery
C. prescribe topical estrogen
D. take a biopsy
E. perform a cryosurgery and prescribe a course of antibiotics

91. The primary difference between smooth muscle and skeletal muscle is that smooth muscle has
A. a lack of stress relaxation
B. a more extensive sarcoplasmic reticulum
C. a smaller ratio of thin to thick filaments
D. a lower velocity of shortening
E. a greater vulnerability to pharmacological agents

92. What part of the nephron is both semipermeable to water and hormonally regulated?
A. ascending loop of Henle
B. Bowman's capsule
C. collecting tubule
D. descending loop of Henle
E. proximal convoluted tubule

93. Oxidation of acetyl-CoA by the enzymes of the citric acid cycle results in the formation of how many moles of ATP for every mole of acetyl-CoA consumed?
A. 6
B. 9
C. 12
D. 14
E. 15

94. A 21-year-old speed skater fell, fracturing the medial epicondyle of the humerus. He lost sensation and flexion ability of the little finger. What other structure was probably damaged?
A. median nerve
B. brachial artery
C. ulnar nerve
D. radial nerve
E. superficial radial nerve

95. You deliver a very sick, large-for-date, ruddy infant with a ventral septal defect. Which of the following most likely describes the mother of this infant?
A. alcoholic
B. cocaine addict
C. diabetic
D. heavy smoker
E. over 45 years of age

96. The term **cardiac afterload** refers to
A. end-diastolic volume effects on the heart
B. aortic pressure against which the heart is contracting

C. atrial filling pressure of the ventricles
D. venous return effects on cardiac output
E. combined effects of all of the above

97. Physical signs characteristic of pure right-sided heart failure include all of the following **except**
A. enlarged tender liver
B. neck vein distention
C. palpable spleen
D. peripheral edema
E. rales on lung auscultation

98. In the theoretical metabolic pathway depicted below, which reaction would be a poor candidate for a control point?
A. A→C
B. B→C
C. C↔D
D. D→E
E. D→F

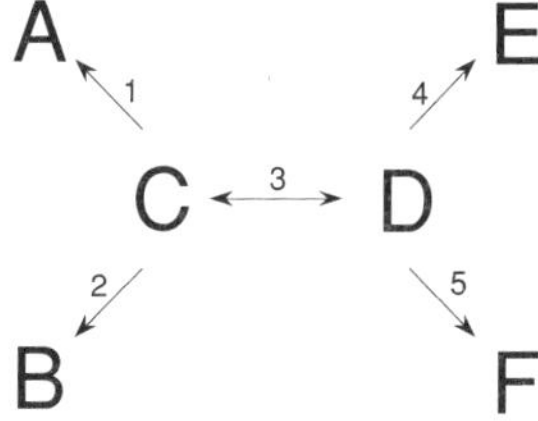

Items 99–102

Match the nuclei listed below with the associated neurotransmitter.

A. dopamine
B. acetylcholine (Ach)
C. histamine
D. norepinephrine
E. seratonin

99. nucleus basalis
100. locus ceruleus
101. substantia nigra
102. midline of the pons

103. Very low density lipoproteins transport
A. nonesterified fatty acids to the liver
B. medium-chain nonesterified fatty acids via the lymph system
C. nonesterified fatty acids to adipose tissue
D. triacylglycerol from the liver to adipose tissue
E. dietary cholesterol to the liver

104. Two weeks after a "cold," a 1-year-old child with no past medical problems presents in the emergency room with acute congestive heart fail-

ure. Chest x-ray reveals an enlarged cardiac silhouette. The most likely diagnosis is
A. acute viral myocarditis
B. cardiac tamponade
C. hypertrophic cardiomyopathy
D. purulent pericarditis
E. undiagnosed congenital heart anomaly

105. Growth hormone administration will lead to all of the following **except**
A. an increase in glucose uptake in fat
B. an increase in gluconeogenesis
C. increased release of IGF-1 from the liver
D. increased amino acid uptake in muscle
E. increased lipolysis in fat

106. In the normal development of a child, the earliest experience of a sense of autonomy occurs during which of the following age ranges?
A. 1–2 years
B. 2–3 years
C. 4–5 years
D. 5–10 years
E. 10–12 years

107. Fasting leads to
A. an increased insulin to glucagon ratio
B. decreased gluconeogenesis
C. increased glycogenesis
D. increased amino acid uptake in muscle
E. None of the above are effects of fasting.

108. Loop diuretics have several side effects, including all of the following **except**
A. hyperuricemia
B. hyperkalemia
C. hypotension
D. ototoxicity
E. exacerbation of gout

109. The reticular nucleus of the thalamus
A. is the center for "intention" and "will"
B. relays nonsensory data to the cortex
C. relays sensory data to the cortex
D. modulates other thalamic nuclei
E. performs all of the above functions

110. According to the cognitive theory, there is an invariable sequence of emerging capacities. Which of the following correctly orders these emerging abilities?

1. Clearly separates objects from self.
2. Recalls objects not in current sight.

3. Eye-following.
4. Symbolic capacity greatly expands.
   A. 3-2-1-4
   B. 4-3-2-1
   C. 3-1-2-4
   D. 3-4-1-2
   E. 3-2-4-1

111. Two drugs are considered to be biologically equivalent. This means that
   A. the two drugs reach equal concentrations in the systemic circulation across the same time span
   B. the two drugs have identical therapeutic effects
   C. the two drugs can be administered using the same dosing regimen
   D. the two drugs reach the same serum and tissue concentrations
   E. one drug may be legally sold as the generic form of the other drug

112. The primary drug used to control the symptoms of Tourette's disorder is
   A. meprobamate
   B. doxepin
   C. haloperidol
   D. imipramine
   E. lithium carbonate

113. The most likely time for drugs or antibodies to cross the placental barrier is
   A. after regression of the capillaries in the fetal membranes
   B. before the formation of the chorionic mesoderm
   C. immediately after regression of the chorionic villi associated with the decidua capsularis
   D. prior to closure of the uterine lumen at midgestation
   E. the last month of the last trimester

114. Vitamin K is involved in blood coagulation in which of the following ways?
   A. It binds to prothrombin, stimulating activation to thrombin.
   B. It competes with dicumarol for a binding site on the platelet membrane.
   C. It is a cofactor for a carboxylase that modifies prothrombin in the propeptide region.
   D. It reacts with factor V, allowing interaction of this factor with the platelet membrane surface.
   E. It is found at the active site of thrombin.

115. Tamoxifen has been found very useful in the treatment of certain cancers of the breast because it can
   A. function as an estrogen antagonist
   B. function as a progestin
   C. block the ovary from producing estrogen
   D. retard tumor growth through its androgenic actions
   E. intensify the effect of glucocorticoid treatment

116. Loss of which of the following nuclei is thought to be associated with the development of Alzheimer's disease?
    A. red nucleus
    B. hypothalamus
    C. caudate nucleus
    D. nucleus basalis
    E. uncus

117. A patient has difficulty in raising the upper eyelid, medial movement of the eyeball, and pupillary dilation. Which cranial nerve most likely is the site of the lesion?
    A. facial (VII)
    B. oculomotor (III)
    C. abducens (VI)
    D. ophthalmic (V1)
    E. trochlear (IV)

Items 118–121

Match each drug or drug category to the appropriate property

A. Blocks dopamine receptors.
B. Can act as hypnotic agent(s).
C. Low therapeutic index.
D. Mechanism of action is unknown.
E. Block(s) reuptake of amine neurotransmitters.

118. tricyclic antidepressants
119. phenothiazines
120. benzodiazepines
121. lithium

122. Which of the following drugs is indicated for the treatment of attention deficit disorder (ADD) in children?
    A. benzodiazepines
    B. theobromine
    C. amphetamine
    D. methylphenidate
    E. nikethamide

123. An increase in plasma colloid osmotic pressure causes
    A. water to move into the tissue
    B. water to move into the blood
    C. no change in capillary fluid balance
    D. a directly proportional change in potassium level
    E. none of the effects described above

124. Platelet aggregation is stimulated by
    A. prostacyclin released from endothelial cells
    B. thromboxane A_2
    C. aspirin

D. increases in cAMP level
E. None of the above is correct.

125. A diabetic smoker comes to the emergency room complaining of cold toes in the right foot. Physical examination reveals normal femoral, posterior tibialis and popliteal pulses but an absent dorsalis pedis pulse. The embolus that is causing his symptoms is likely to be lodged in the
A. peroneal artery
B. anterior tibial artery
C. femoral artery
D. posterior tibial artery
E. popliteal artery

126. Which of the following is most likely to cause congenital malformations when transmitted from mother to fetus during the first trimester?
A. erythema infectiosum
B. roseola infantum
C. rubella
D. rubeola
E. variola

127. Increased levels of motor activity might be expected in patients who suffer from all of the following disorders **except**
A. lesions of the nigrostriatal tract
B. attention deficit disorders
C. tardive dyskinesia
D. mania
E. delirium

128. Identify the potassium-sparing diuretic in the following group:
A. acetazolamide
B. bumetanide
C. chlorothiazide
D. ethacrynic acid
E. triamterene

129. Of the following, the **least likely** cause of acute right lower quadrant pain in a 25-year-old sexually active woman is
A. acute appendicitis
B. acute salpingitis
C. adenocarcinoma of the cecum with perforation
D. Crohn's disease of the terminal ileum
E. ectopic (tubal) pregnancy

130. Which of the following actions would be an example of H_1-receptor antagonist toxicity?
A. dry mouth
B. constipation
C. itching
D. hyperpyrexia
E. sedation

131. Identify the muscle pair that **is not** mutually antagonistic.
   A. gluteus minimus–adductor longus
   B. iliopsoas–gluteus maximus
   C. obturator externus–gluteus minimus
   D. iliopsoas–rectus femoris
   E. piriformis–gluteus medius

Items 132–134

Match each response to death with the appropriate stage of the life cycle. Each choice may be used once, more than once, or not at all.

A. age 2–5 years
B. age 6–10 years
C. age 11–13 years
D. age 30–40 years
E. 75 years and older

132. The terminally ill person fears dying before having "left his mark" on the world.
133. The deceased person is perceived as having abandoned everyone.
134. The survivor feels punished for bad behavior by the death of the loved one.

Items 135–137

For each question, select the organism most closely associated with it.

A. adenovirus
B. coronavirus
C. cytomegalovirus
D. hepatitis A virus
E. hepatitis B virus
F. herpes simplex virus type 1
G. mumps virus
H. parainfluenza virus type 1
I. rabies virus
J. respiratory syncytia virus type 1
K. retrovirus
L. rhinovirus
M. vaccinia virus
N. western equine encephalitis virus

135. A 14-month-old boy was seen at a clinic in October after development of a fever and barking cough that had persisted for 3 days. His throat was red and the upper respiratory tract was congested, but no evidence of pneumonia was found. Virus was cultured from nasopharyngeal specimens and identified by hemadsorption. What is the most likely etiologic agent?
136. Viremia usually occurs following infections with this organism.
137. A helical capsid surrounded by an envelope derived from cellular membrane is characteristic of this organism.

Items 138–141

A. amikacin
B. bacitracin
C. chloramphenicol
D. erythromycin
I. neomycin
J. penicillin G
K. piperacillin
L. streptomycin

E. gentamicin
F. kanamycin
G. lincomycin
H. nafcillin
M. tetracycline
N. tobramycin
O. vancomycin

138. Because of an outbreak of *Legionella* pneumonia, the clinic ran short of this drug.
139. This is the most effective antimicrobial agent against infections caused by *Pseudomonas aeruginosa*.
140. A certain organism shows resistance to gentamicin. You would most likely try this agent as an effective alternate aminoglycoside.
141. This is the drug of choice for treating cases of *Mycoplasma pneumoniae* since the organism has no cell wall.

Items 142–145

Match each organism with its characteristic vector.

A. tick and flea bites
B. ingestion of contaminated food
C. contact with animal urine
D. shared eating utensils
E. insect vectors such as flies
F. bites of lice
G. infected rodents
H. nasopharyngeal tract of cats
I. direct human-to-human contact

142. leptospirosis
143. epidemic relapsing fever
144. Lyme disease
145. whooping cough

Items 146–150

Match each description with the nerve or artery with which it is most closely associated.

A. anterior cerebral artery
B. basilar artery
C. facial nerve
D. glossopharyngeal nerve
E. hypoglossal nerve
F. internal carotid artery
G. mandibular nerve
H. middle cerebral artery
I. vagus nerve
J. vertebral artery

146. Innervates pharyngeal motor muscles.
147. A branch of this artery supplies the eyeball.
148. Supplies the thalamus and basal ganglia.
149. Taste fibers to the anterior two thirds of the tongue.
150. Supplies the inferior cerebellum.

Answers for the Diagnostic Pretest

1. D
2. B
3. A
4. A
5. D
6. C
7. C
8. D
9. D

10. C
11. C
12. E
13. A
14. A
15. C
16. B
17. C
18. A
19. D
20. B
21. E
22. D
23. E
24. B
25. E
26. B
27. C
28. D
29. E
30. B
31. A
32. C
33. D
34. C
35. D
36. E
37. A
38. D
39. C
40. D
41. D
42. E
43. B
44. C
45. D
46. E
47. C
48. E
49. D
50. B
51. B
52. A
53. E
54. E
55. D
56. E
57. D
58. B
59. E
60. E
61. B
62. E
63. D
64. A
65. E
66. E
67. B
68. E
69. D
70. A
71. E
72. C
73. C
74. B
75. D
76. C
77. D
78. B
79. A
80. E
81. A
82. B
83. C
84. B
85. B
86. D
87. C
88. D
89. E
90. D
91. D
92. C
93. C
94. C
95. C
96. B
97. E
98. C
99. B
100. D
101. A
102. E
103. D
104. A
105. A
106. B
107. E
108. B
109. D
110. A
111. D
112. C
113. E
114. C
115. B
116. D
117. B
118. E
119. A
120. B
121. D
122. D
123. B
124. B
125. B
126. C
127. A
128. E
129. C
130. D
131. D
132. D
133. A
134. B
135. H
136. G
137. H
138. C
139. K
140. A
141. M
142. C
143. F
144. A
145. I
146. I
147. F
148. H
149. C
150. J

2

Test-Taking and Study Skills

Preparing for the Boards

Preparing for the USMLE Step 1 examination won't feel nearly as overwhelming if you approach the task with a carefully prepared strategy for making the most of your time and resources. In a sense, you began the preparation process during basic science courses taken in the first year of medical school. This is especially true if you found it necessary and helpful to make condensed notes, charts, or summaries as you prepared for course examinations. These abbreviated versions of the central content of course material are valuable jewels in your review process that you have already prepared. Because **you** prepared them, they helped you learn and retain the material better at the time. Now, as you plan how you will review for each subject area, they can be fitted into your review process and will serve that process far more efficiently than a newly purchased review book because their style and organization are your own—they match the way you viewed and learned the material in the first place. Therefore, as a first step in planning your review, take stock of any content summaries you have for each course so that you can use them, when possible, instead of new review materials.

A systematic review plan that follows a regular schedule is important if you are going to make the best use of the time you have for reviewing. Three general organizational strategies are presented here for you to consider as you plan: (1) reviewing by organ system, (2) reviewing by subject area, and (3) reviewing by linking review topics to a current pathology course syllabus. Each strategy has associated disadvantages as well as advantages. You should select a plan that fits your own style of studying and feels most comfortable or logical to you. However, be aware that the USMLE Step 1 stresses clinical material and therefore contains many questions that address multisystemic processes in healthy and diseased states. Many students reported that they found it difficult to tell what subject area a given item was testing because it focused on an area of overlap between two subjects. Items that assess molecular genetics or mechanisms of autoimmune disorders would be typical examples. These topics fall between traditional divisions of basic science disciplines yet are on the cutting edge of current medical research. In fact, it is a good idea for you to pay special attention to topics that overlap several basic science areas since they are likely to be tested fairly intensively on Step 1.

We return to our discussion of overall review strategies by explaining how each one works. Reviewing by organ system has become increasingly popular since the USMLE Step 1 examination was phased in. By its very nature, this approach is cross-disciplinary and can therefore help students who are attending schools that teach by the traditional subject areas of anatomy, physiology, pathology, and so on. While there is nothing wrong with learning basic science material in this way, it can be a slight disadvantage when students review for Step 1 because the material is organized in memory by these subject divisions. While most students try to relate what they learn about the structure of the kidney in anatomy to its filtering mechanisms, which are learned in physiology, the pace and volume pressures on most students make such integration incomplete at best.

Reviewing by organ systems can help you make connections so that your understanding is better integrated, and organized in memory in a way that will serve you better as you begin clinical rotations. After all, the attending physicians who will be working with you in the hospitals aren't going to ask you about the capsule structure of *Neisseria*, but they are more likely to say, "So you think this lady has an infection. What type of specimen are you going to collect and how do you want it cultured?" As you can see, it is important to be able to integrate what you know, not just to do well on Step 1, but also to begin to apply what you know to clinical situations, to real patients' problems.

An organ system review involves sequentially reviewing the chapters in various subject-bound review books that cover a specific organ. For example, you might start by reviewing the anatomy of the respiratory system; move to respiratory physiology; look at the bacterial, viral, and fungal agents that produce respiratory infections; then move on to respiratory pathology; and end with a review of the pharmacological approaches to treating asthma, pneumonia, tuberculosis, COPD, and so forth. This review sequence has a number of advantages. One is the sense of momentum you will feel as you move, at first slowly through the anatomy and physiology you studied the first year, and then more quickly, as you move on to the microbiology, pathology, and pharmacology that you studied very recently. Another advantage is the fact that if you feel weak in a particular basic science subject or actually dislike it, your review time in the area will be cut into briefer sessions, interspersed among five or six other subjects' perspectives on the particular organ system you are reviewing. In fact, you may actually begin to understand the disliked or weaker area better as you see its relationship to the other disciplines.

A review plan that mixes reviewing by organ system with subject-based reviews of material that doesn't lend itself to organ-based reviewing is shown in Figure 2-1. Notice that this review plan begins with a series of topics that covers aspects of medical science at the process or molecular levels. These topics should be placed at the beginning because they deal with central mechanisms that underlie all organ system functioning. The section is therefore labelled "introductory." You will find these topics in the early sections of specific review books. As you finish a particular review topic, you could keep track by simply crossing that chapter off in the table of contents of the individual review book to keep track of where you are on the plan. The second section of the mixed review plan is the "systemic review." To some degree, the organ systems are grouped in order of importance. Major systems such as cardiovascular, renal, and respiratory are listed first. Less heavily tested systems such as skin/breast are listed last. This is done to ensure that if time runs short, you will have covered the most important systems most thoroughly and given the lesser systems a more cursory look.

The final section of the mixed review plan contains the topics that are not

Topics	**Sources (books, notes, etc.)**
Introductory	
Cell biology	
Membrane physiology	
Inflammation and repair	
Pharmacokinetics	
Systemic review	
Cardiovascular	
Respiratory	
Renal	
Nervous system	
Central	
Peripheral	
Genitourinary	
Gastrointestinal	
Hepatic	
Endocrine	
Musculoskeletal	
Special senses	
Skin/breast	
Subject-based review	
Biochemistry	
Microbiology	
Behavioral sciences	

Fig. 2-1. One example of a mixed review plan.

easily integrated into systems. Thus, biochemistry and behavioral sciences stand alone. Microbiology can be integrated or can be covered separately, depending on the review materials you select and how this material was taught at your school. Because so many courses in microbiology in medical schools organize the material into bacteriology, virology, and fungi rather than by the medical problems caused by the organisms, it is often easier to review this area as a separate subject than to locate the various pieces that relate to heart, kidney, or lung.

The order in which topics are covered is an important consideration in any review strategy. Material that deals with mechanisms and processes can be reviewed earlier because that type of content tends to be retained longer in memory. More rote material such as structural aspects of bacteria or biochemical pathways is more quickly forgotten and therefore should be reviewed closer to the time of examination. You can now understand why microbiology and biochemistry are shown in the final "subject-based review" section of the mixed review plan. The final area to be discussed is behavioral sciences. This is a very broad, eclectic area on Step 1. It includes normal human psychological development in addition to abnormal behavior, behavioral correlates of human disease, and cultural risk factors, as well as concepts in biostatistics and epidemiology. Most students find reviewing this kind of material to be a welcome relief from the "harder" science areas. Rather than setting aside specific times to review it, they slip its topics in among other basic science topics as a welcome change of pace.

It is relatively easy to keep track of where you stand in the mixed review plan by either marking off chapters completed in the various review books used during the systemic review section or by using a sheet such as the one shown in Figure 2-1. You may wonder why so many review books have organ-based chapter organization. The answer is simple: The authors hope to be able to sell books at schools that use traditional or organ-based curricula, and, therefore, while most review materials are produced in separate volumes by subject, the chapter organization is by organ system.

The second review strategy is the subject-based review plan. In this strategy, you would review anatomy, physiology, then biochemistry, and so on until you have completed all the major areas studied in the basic science years. It would be very helpful to have a topic matrix to follow within each subject, such as the one provided in the USMLE Step 1 *General Instructions, Content Description, and Sample Items* booklet. You will receive one of these booklets from your medical school when you register to take Step 1.

A time plan for reviewing each subject area is still important, since you will want to allow the **most** time to your **weakest** areas and the **least** time to your **strongest** areas. The general rule for allotting time to review areas is to put the most time into your gaps, making your profile as even as possible. It is never safe to write off a significant content area simply because you reason that you are weak in it and therefore probably won't do well, instead putting time into an area in which you are very strong and thus hoping to be able to make up those lost points. This strategy can spell disaster on Step 1. Why? Because you have to compete against the entire population taking the exam on the stronger area in order to make up the points lost in the "written-off" area.

In the subject-based plan, you will still need to think about how much time to allow for review in each area. This decision should be based on the general principle of using less time for your strengths and more time for your weak areas. You should also reserve a few days at the very end to go over the more rote memorization aspects of each subject, such as pathways, mathematical formulas, and so forth.

The final review strategy is called the pathology-based strategy because it utilizes the sequence of topics in your medical school pathology course to sequence reviewing. It is somewhat similar to the organ-based plan in that selected aspects of all areas are reviewed as they apply to particular pathologic states or mechanisms of disease. One example of such a review plan is shown in Figure 2-2. For each disease cluster or category, you would be reviewing to answer questions such as the following ones pertaining to a particular tumor: Where is it located and why does it locate there? What is the pharmacology of this tumor? What is its biochemistry? How does its structure deviate from that of normal tissue? How does its diagnosis/treatment/prognosis compare to that of other tumors? Since questions like these are fairly generic, they can be posed repeatedly for one topic after another. The point of using questions is that they help make your review process a more mentally active one. You will tend to retain more information when you read to answer a question than if you read simply with the intent to "cover" a certain topic.

Some people find it very difficult to create review questions like those described for themselves. If this is a problem for you, relax. Review materials nearly always include ample numbers of questions for practice and these can be used to give your review reading a concrete purpose. Using questions **before** reviewing material is the key to efficient review. The items provide you with a method for determining your current level of recall so you will know where to concentrate your time and effort. Prereview self-testing helps you sort your knowledge into three broad categories: (1) "know-it-cold" material, (2) "hazy-understanding" material, and (3) material about which you are

Topics	Sources (books, notes, etc.)
General pathology	
Pathology of the cell	
Inflammation and repair mechanisms	
Diseases caused by physical, chemical agents	
Environmental diseases	
Radiation effects	
Nutritional diseases	
Degenerative processes	
Aging	
Homeostasis, shock, and heart failure	
Infarction, thrombosis, and embolism	
Neoplasia	
Congenital and genetic disorders	
Immunopathology	
Infectious disease	
Systemic pathology	
Respiratory pathology	
Cardiovascular pathology	
Renal/male urogenital pathology	
Endocrine pathology	
Skin pathology	
Breast pathology	
Special senses disorders	
Alimentary pathology	
Hepatobiliary pathology	
Female genital system and pregnancy disorders	
Diseases of soft tissue and muscle	
Diseases of bone and joints	
Hematology	
Neuropathology	
Diseases of childhood	

Fig. 2-2. One example of a pathology-based review plan.

"clueless." While the limited time you have will probably make it impossible to attempt to learn material in the third category, your review process should aim at clarifying the hazy material and refreshing your recall of the material you know very well.

Using questions for practice throughout the review process has a number of significant advantages. In addition to helping you decide where to spend review time, question sessions offer a welcome change of pace from the mind-numbing aspects of review reading. Questions keep you honest with yourself. It's common for people to assume they know certain material when what's really true is that the material sounds familiar and they can recognize the important aspects within the material as they read it. This is very different from the "knowing" that allows you to actively recall specifics during an exam in response to a particular test item. Finally, question sessions allow you to hone your test-taking skills, and to practice interpreting questions and arriving at educated guesses.

It is wise to practice in the mode that most closely matches the actual test. In this case, multiple-choice questions on basic science topics are the closest mimic. In fact, if you have the opportunity, you might want to sign up to take a simulated USMLE Step 1 examination a month or two before the real test date so that you will know exactly what to expect and how to pace yourself to finish in the allotted time for each booklet. If your school does not offer a simulation, several practice tests are available in medical bookstores that you can purchase and take on your own. Each has directions for mimicking the

USMLE test conditions and at least one offers a computer-generated diagnostic profile of your performance.

Self-Evaluation of Current Skills Through Error Analysis

If you have ever run into significant problems on tests for a course in medical school or college although you felt you understood the material and had prepared well for the exams, you are already familiar with that feeling of not being in control of your own learning. This feeling can bring on even more test errors, as your self-confidence decreases and you begin to second-guess your answers on item after item. In the worst-case scenario, the problem grows until you begin to dread the next exam and lose sleep over the prospect of yet another period of intense study followed by disappointing results.

Most people struggle to master material sooner or later. No matter how intelligent we think we are, there may come a time when the material initially confuses us or the work load prohibits mastery of the material to our own internal standards of excellence. The prospect of preparing for the USMLE Step 1 can accentuate the problem. Anxiety is perfectly normal in test-taking situations, but if you reach a point where you don't even know where to begin and feel defeated before you start, you need to take control and meet the problem head-on.

One of the most common complaints that I hear from medical students is that they don't do as well on exams as their classmates, even though they know the material just as well. This may sound like rationalization, but it isn't. It is very possible for two students to have approximately the same amount of knowledge about a topic and yet one student does significantly better on the exam. The reason for the difference in apparent knowledge is test-taking skill. Many of you probably know someone who always seems to be able to make the right educated guesses when he or she is not sure of the answer by means of recalled information alone. Is this just a matter of luck or something more?

Luck or, rather, probability can play a role in guessing correctly on test questions. In most cases, however, lucky "guesses" are actually based on more than chance. They often flow from a thought process making use of subtle cues present in the test question, the format of the question, or even the general nature of the material being assessed by the question. Later in this chapter, you will be shown how to use these cues to make better answer choices on tests.

First, I want you to examine how you currently take tests. I call the process of systematically scrutinizing your test errors "error analysis." You are going to use the process to look at your performance on the Diagnostic Pretest. The objective of this error analysis is to determine whether you have any test-taking or study habits that are resulting in errors on material that you do, in fact, know.

Figure 2-3 illustrates an error analysis worksheet. Figure 2-4 provides an example of a hypothetical student's analysis so that we can examine it together. By looking at this student's errors (we'll call the student Sam), you will have an easier time interpreting any error patterns that you might find in your own performance. First, however, you need to learn how to perform the

Item#	Format	Item descriptor	Task/process

Fig. 2-3. Error analysis worksheet.

error analysis itself. Then you can read the discussion on the example with a better understanding of how to use the data on your own errors.

The error analysis form uses a number of vertical columns to record information about each item answered incorrectly. The column farthest to the left is labelled "item #." Use it to record the number of any item you missed in the Diagnostic Pretest. Leave enough space between item numbers so that you will have room to write a brief phrase or two under any column (about 1/2 in. should be enough).

The second column is labelled "format." In this column, record your own abbreviations for the various types of questions used. I use SBA for the standard single best answer items. Those matching items with the long lists of possible responses I call EXM, which is shorthand for extended matching items. Proceed until you have recorded all your errors and categorized them by format.

The third column is labelled "item descriptor." This column is used to record a brief description of the topic and essential aspects of each question. It will take you a little while to feel comfortable doing this, but it is absolutely necessary to record a meaningful descriptor for every item missed. It might help to look at the descriptors for some of Sam's errors in Figure 2-4. With a little

Fig. 2-4. Sam's error analysis worksheet.

Item#	Format	Item descriptor	Task/process
5	SBA	Biostatistics	Calculate mean
11	SBA	Pharmacokinetics	Calculate pKa
13	Neg. SBA	ID incorrect stmt.: child abuse	Discr. false stmt.
14	Neg. SBA	Synthet. products–liver	Discr. false stmt.
24	Neg. SBA	Nl vs. abnl. grieving	Discr. false stmt.
38	Neg. SBA	Dxs if ↑ HCG	Discr. false stmt.
43	Matching	Defense mech.	Definition
44	Matching	Defense mech.	Definition
46	Neg. SBA	Lab tech using antibodies	Discr. false stmt.
61	SBA	Carcinoma characteristics	Definition
80	SBA	Pathologic fractures	Definition

Summary: Overall % correct = 66%
Overall error rate = 44%

Neg. items: 60% error rate
Definitions: 55% error rate
Math. calcs: 50% error rate

practice, you will be able to generate a brief descriptor for any type of item in no time.

The final column is labelled "task/process." This column is used to note the demands that each item made on you as you attempted to answer it. These notes should capture a little more than just the topic of the question. Some people like to think about the task/process column entries in terms of what a test taker has to be able to do mentally in order to get an item correct. An item assessing the differences between skeletal and cardiac muscle cells, for example, might require the test taker to be able to identify structural features that are only present in cardiac tissue and not in skeletal muscle cells. Knowing the shared features, then, might not be sufficient to answer the question correctly. The "task" notation for such an item might read "CC: ID unique features of cardiac m. cells (vs. skel.)." CC is an abbreviation for compare and contrast items, ID is short for the task of identifying. Once again, if you are not sure what to say about an item, scan the error analysis of our friend Sam to see what he recorded for specific items in the Diagnostic Pretest to get a better feel for the task. Fill in an appropriate task notation for each item on your error analysis worksheet now.

Error analysis usually takes about a minute per question to complete and the information potential of the product may be worth a great deal in helping you improve your performance on standardized and even faculty-generated tests. Just as in the practice of clinical medicine, however, you must take the time to arrive at a careful diagnosis before you can begin to treat a problem effectively.

Interpreting Your Error Analysis

Now that you have filled in the form completely, you are going to analyze the data to determine whether there are patterns among the items you missed. To give you a clearer picture of how to do this, let's look again at Sam's error patterns in Figure 2-4.

Here is a summary of the patterns found in Sam's errors: First, Sam made a disproportionate number of errors on items that were negatively phrased. These are items such as numbers 13 and 14 on the Diagnostic Pretest. We know that Sam had a higher error rate on these by comparing how he fared on the total test (66% correct or 44% error rate overall) to how he did on negatively phrased items. His error rate on the negative items was 60% over the total test, which means that he missed 2 of 3 items with this format. This finding may lead Sam to pay more attention to exceptions to a general rule when he reviews material for Step 1. Now that Sam sees how much worse he does on these items, he can take steps to correct the problem.

The second error pattern involves items that dealt with definitions of terms, especially in the behavioral sciences. Examples of such items include numbers 42 through 45 and number 77. Since Sam clearly missed a large number of items assessing this subject, it is a generally weak area into which he will have to put more time. There may be a second problem in that Sam may habitually understudy definitions. Many students form subtle habits that cause problems as they move into new courses and subjects in which new emphases demand adjustments in deciding what is most important to study. Sam might want to look at his last few exams to see if he missed quite a few definition items there, too. If so, he can make an effort to lock in his knowledge of key definitions as he reviews in order to avoid losing any more points to this unconscious habit.

The final pattern may not reflect a real pattern in Sam at all. Notice that Sam missed a number of questions involving mathematical concepts and calculations. Depending on when Sam took the Pretest, this may simply reflect the fact that the material assessed in these items was learned first and hasn't yet been reviewed. Certainly Sam would be in a position to assess whether he has a weakness in this area and, if so, he will need to find practice items to work with until he feels confident that items that require formulas or graph interpretation won't be a problem on Step 1.

As you can see from the above discussion, analyzing errors is suggestive rather than definitive. You look at the data to see what they suggest, and then you must use your own judgment to determine whether you are seeing evidence of an actual test-taking problem or merely an artifact. You are the best judge. Here is a summary of some common error patterns and how to check for them. If you think you see a pattern in your errors, refer to this summary, which also offers a few suggestions on how to "treat" the problem. If a definite pattern is found, be sure to do an error analysis of your performance on the Posttest at the end of this book. You should see fewer errors overall and, if you have taken whatever patterns you found seriously and tried to remedy them, fewer errors of that type as well.

Common Error Patterns

Format Patterns

To determine whether a particular format of question is problematic, you will have to calculate an error rate for each of the formats used on the exam. Only four test formats are used in this book because they reflect the formats used on Step 1. The formats include single best answer, single best answer **except**, matching with five choices, and extended matching with more than five choices. You may find it helpful to separate items that entail math or graph interpretation as a separate category if these appear to be a problem.

For each format, count the number of items in this format on the exam. Count the number you missed in the format. Divide the number missed by the total number to get your error rate for that format. Compare this error rate to your overall error rate. Your overall error rate is just 100% minus the percent you got right on the exam. For example, if you scored 62% correct overall, your overall error rate is 100 – 62, or 38%. Now you can compare your error rates across all four test formats. If the variation is within 10 to 15% of your overall rate, you probably don't have to worry about a format pattern.

Test Anxiety Patterns

You are less likely to discover evidence of test anxiety when you are taking a test for practice because you will be more relaxed. After all, the score won't affect your grade and there is usually less time pressure than in an actual test situation. Some people find *any* test situation threatening. Each error is seen as more evidence that they are not going to pass, that they don't "have what it takes." In any event, it is important to look at your performance carefully if you believe that test anxiety has been affecting your performance. This is how to check for evidence of such a problem.

Examine the first 50 items on the Diagnostic Pretest. Is your error rate quite a bit higher than it was on the total test? If it was higher, you may have a problem that is most likely to affect your thought process and recall *early* in an exam. Once you have settled down to the task and psychologically composed yourself, there is less chance of missing items, which is why the error rate goes down later in the exam.

In some cases of test anxiety or emotional overreaction to the test situation, the problem surfaces later in the exam. This is especially evident if the test taker encounters a cluster of difficult items and temporarily loses confidence. There is a significant probability of making "dumb" mistakes just after the problematic group of items, because the test taker is still dealing with those emotions and is not concentrating as fully on the subsequent questions.

A similar pattern of apparently "silly" mistakes can occur just following an item that triggers anger in the test taker. Have you ever been assured by a lecturer that a certain topic would not be tested, that it was being discussed "simply for your information," and then seen an item or two on that topic show up on the next test? When this happens, most test takers feel tricked and upset. Items that are worded in a confusing or needlessly wordy fashion trigger anger, too. Nearly every time test takers allow themselves to become really angry in response to such items, they will be prone to making mistakes that, in retrospect, they can't understand. "How could I have put answer 'C' when the answer is so obviously 'E'?" The students have just paid the price of allowing anger to disrupt their concentration during an exam. The only real defense is self-control. This is easier to achieve when error analysis provides proof of the price paid for getting angry, namely, easy items missed!

Fatigue Pattern

If you examine the last 50 items on the Diagnostic Pretest and compare your error rate on this group versus the total test, you can check for evidence of test-taking fatigue. Again, this is a less likely phenomenon in a self-administered practice situation. On formal exams, students are much more likely to have stayed up late or even all night in order to cram in just a few more hours of study. Having done so, they may never realize the number of errors they will make due to fatigue. Scrutinizing your own exam performance for this pattern requires judgment and being honest with yourself. You might suspect that some of the mistakes you now feel were "stupid" or careless may actually be due to the state of alertness you had as you came to the items on the test day. You may even have held up pretty well throughout most of the test period, but found it very difficult to recall or concentrate on the last few pages of the test. As with several of the error patterns we have discussed, recognizing the problem can go a long way toward solving it. Remembering that you missed three or four items on the last exam because you were exhausted may help you decide the next time that an extra 3 or 4 hours of sleep will probably serve you better than the last few facts you might cram into your tired brain during that same period of time. At least now you have information and can make a more informed decision about the relative benefits of adequate sleep versus an all-night cram session.

Reading Errors

Reading errors are fairly common during exams. You should suspect a reading error if, on careful re-reading of an item, it is obvious that a different answer was called for. You are also more likely to make reading errors on certain types of items. Long, clinical vignette items can cause problems because there is a greater tendency to forget a crucial piece of data when you finally get to the stage of evaluating specific response choices. Negatively phrased questions can be misread, too, if you feel pressed for time or forget, after reading and evaluating several responses, that you are looking for the one that **is not** true. In working with students to improve their test-taking skills, I often have them read and work through items aloud. Frequently, they will verbally delete prefixes, reading "nonmalignant" as "malignant," for example. In other cases, I will stop the student and ask for a paraphrase of the question in the student's own words. During an exam, a student might press on to try to solve the question before fully clarifying his or her understanding of what is being asked. These are all reading errors, and they all cost points, not because of a lack of knowledge, but because the test taker is unaware of test-taking behaviors that are lowering his or her performance.

Directionality Errors

Test items frequently ask for recalled information in an order that is the reverse of the order in which something was learned. In a subject such as physiology, for example, it is common to ask for the step that precedes the one described in the stem of the question. In other cases, the item calls for predicting consequences, such as an item that asks which variables in heart function will be increased when there is a significant loss of blood. Any mechanism or process can be assessed in this manner. The error pattern to look for is a significantly higher error rate of items that assess understanding of mechanisms, those that deal with steps in a process or those that call for determining causes and effects. If a directionality error pattern is found, you can take care to focus on the dynamic aspects during review using simple diagrams or by practicing on questions such as those mentioned above.

Group Delineation Errors

In a sense, this category is the opposite of negatively phrased items. Negative items ask you to identify something that **does not** have certain features or functions. Group delineation items ask you to identify the features or functions that **are common** to a certain group. A group of viruses, childhood diseases, lower socioeconomic group, ethnic minorities in the US, diuretic drugs—almost any grouping you can think of—can be the topic of a question of this form. The error pattern will be higher on items that ask for the common features of the group, usually because the test taker has not looked at the patterns among the specific group members that he or she reviewed. Wouldn't it be easier, for example, to recall which member(s) of a bacterial family had a particular type of capsule structure if one reviewed a chart of that **family** of bacteria that compared the members by their structure, drug sensitivity, vectors, life cycle, and so forth? In this way, you would have **seen** the pattern and perhaps recalled that all but two of the bacteria shared a common feature in capsule structure. This is a clear illustration of the strong link between how you study and review information and how you fare on test questions.

My favorite example of this phenomenon in which we "know" something yet perform well or poorly in situations in which we must use the information concerns the alphabet. All of us can recite the alphabet rapidly, without even really thinking about what letter follows what. Yet if I were to ask you to recite the alphabet backwards, it would be a fairly slow and challenging process. To which you might reply, "Yes, but no one needs to know the alphabet backwards so I never learned it that way." Exactly correct. Now, count backwards from 100 as fast as you can. Surprised at how well you can do this apparently similar task? The difference lies in the way we need to **use** information. Once we realize that test items can take a certain slant on material, we can make intelligent choices about how we need to look at, organize, or review that material so we will feel comfortable looking at the material from that angle, too. Remember, we are only looking to see if your performance shows any strongly suggestive error patterns. If your errors are spread over items that don't seem to share any particular features, then there are no special changes you need to consider in planning your review for Step 1 or in your approach to certain types of items.

Changing Answers

Tally any items where it is evident that you changed an answer (pencil erasures are usually the tip off). Notice that for this analysis, you need to scan **every** item, not just those on which you made errors. Tally the following categories:

1. Wrong to wrong
2. Wrong to right
3. Right to wrong

Disregard the first category. This represents items for which you simply didn't know the material. If category 2 has the largest count, congratulate yourself and skip the rest of this section. You are already an expert at knowing when to change and when not to change answers! If category 3 is the largest, you will make fewer errors if you adopt a very simple rule and follow it strictly. The rule is: I will only change an answer if (A) I find that on re-reading an item, **I actually misread it the first time**, or (B) I later recalled information **specific to that question** that changed my judgment about the correct answer.

This section has presented you with a technique for analyzing your test errors. If you discover a pattern among the errors you made, you can make a specific change in your approach either to test taking or reviewing to lessen the number of errors of that type. As you can now see, simply looking at your total score, or even looking at how you performed on one topic compared to another, does little to reveal what was really going on as you took that test. By thinking systematically about what your errors reveal about your learning and test-taking habits, you can act directly to change your performance. After all, taking tests is supposed to provide you with feedback about your own learning. Test errors can tell you a great deal about **how** you learn, not just **how much** you apparently learned about the subject.

A no-PANIC Approach to Taking Tests

Anxiety is an extremely common student response to taking examinations. What if I didn't study enough to pass? What if I studied the wrong material? What will happen to my grade if I fail? Will I run out of time to finish the exam? While such thoughts are common and an understandable response to the stress of facing an important exam, these negative thoughts can hurt your test performance by distracting you from concentrating on the content of the exam. Encountering a few tough questions in a row can send you into a mental slurry of fear and drooping self-confidence, making it harder to deal with subsequent questions. A long, complicated-sounding question can lead to a rapid "I give up" reaction, followed by a wild guess and, as a consequence, little chance of selecting the correct answer for that item.

The USMLE Step 1 is an important exam. Your score on the test can affect your competitiveness for a residency position in certain medical specialties. In many medical schools, you are required to pass Step 1 in order to continue into the clinical years of your training. With all this riding on how well you do, is it possible to approach the test calmly and with confidence? The answer is a resounding **yes!** This section will show you how to develop a systematic approach to Step 1 and how to "hang in there" throughout all four test periods of the 2-day, 12-hour exam. You will need to practice the various components of this approach as you review over the coming months or weeks in order to make the approach automatic. Once the components feel comfortable, however, you will be able to devote more of your mental capacity to the content matter of each question. This, in turn, will lead to fewer careless errors and a better overall use of time. In short, adopting the no-PANIC approach will enhance your test-taking ability.

Each capitalized letter in the no-PANIC approach stands for an activity in which you should engage during the test. This simple mnemonic device should make the steps easier for you to remember, even when you are feeling those familiar test-day jitters. Here is an explanation of each part of the approach.

P Stands for Pacing

Standardized examinations nearly always impose strict time limitations. Before you are allowed to break the seal of a test booklet, the time allowed is usually announced, and remaining time is also announced in hourly or half-hourly increments. Don't rely on these verbal announcements to gauge your time use. You must take charge of your own pacing. Have a plan for time use in mind before you start and stick to the plan. Here is an example of a pacing plan:

- Each Step 1 booklet contains 200 items. I am allowed 3 hours per booklet. This means I have approximately 55 seconds for answering each item.
- I always like to return to a few items to check my work, but my error analysis showed that I tend to lose points by changing from right to wrong answers. So I will try to use all of the allowed time as I proceed through the booklet and not let myself rethink any answers. I'll allow some time leeway at the end by trying to pace myself at 50 seconds per item, just in case I run a little long on some questions.
- When I open the booklet, I'll flip to items numbers 50, 100, and 150, and put a big star in the margin next to them. I'll check my time only when I come to these marked items so I won't break my concentration all the time by checking my watch or the clock.

As you can see, this student is taking charge of the test situation. Information from his own error analysis is used to decide what strategy makes the most sense, given his habit of second-guessing himself and changing answers. By premarking the items one quarter, one half, and three quarters of the way through the total test booklet, he is imposing a pacing system that will allow him to adjust his time appropriately, yet not break his concentration by repeatedly checking his watch out of sheer nervousness. Even before he begins answering items, he is in control of the time factor.

A second pacing strategy is necessary for making the best use of time during Step 1. You need to make a conscious decision about handling different types of items. As you practice with questions during the review process, be alert to the kinds of questions that seem to call for recall alone. Such items are frequently the type that ask which nerve, drug, or bug has X or Y feature. Little information is given in the item for you to think or reason with, and you can usually tell fairly quickly that this particular item is going to be one for which you simply know the answer or you don't.

Practice recognizing items like the ones described above quickly. Have a guessing rule and invoke it when you don't know the answer. Your guessing rule might be simply to answer "C" to all such items. It doesn't particularly matter what rule you choose, but invoking the rule when the item doesn't lend itself to reasoning strategies keeps you from wasting valuable time during the exam by trying to decide which answer to select when you don't really have any information on which to base a decision. If this makes you nervous, remember that you can miss a fair number of items on Step 1 and still do very well. If you allow yourself to waste time on items when you have a very low probability of "figuring out" a correct answer, however, you won't have the time to think through many other items for which you have a much better chance of making a correct, educated guess.

Pacing for Step 1 also involves what you do in the last day before the exam. This is not a time to drive yourself to distraction by cramming in a last-minute barrage of detailed information. In fact, learning research has shown that information looked at just before a test can actually interfere with recall of information learned earlier. The day before is a time to spend in pleasant, noncognitive activities. Swim, jog, see a good movie. Rest your mind and body so they will perform well for you over the next 2 days.

If you have problems sleeping before big exams, try to engage in an activity that leaves you physically spent. Try not to socialize with anyone who is taking Step 1 unless he or she knows enough to leave the topic alone. Panic is a communicable disease!

A Stands for Analyzing

After you open the test booklet, allow yourself the time to look through the booklet to see how the items with the same format are arranged. Are all the extended matching questions grouped together? Does the booklet have the usual number of items? Is there some white space in the page margins or at the end of the test booklet that you can use to jot down important formulas, useful mnemonics, or diagrams that you are sure to need to answer more than just a single item? Where is the table of normal values and which values are given in it? Do you want to jot down a few more so they'll be there if and when they're needed?

While it may seem strange to spend a minute or two surveying the test booklet in this manner, it is very important. Do it to set the right tone for the whole day. Psychologically, this brief survey of what you must deal with helps you settle in to the test-taking task. By jotting a few items you think you might need later, you are warming up the retrieval process and relieving yourself of the fear that you might not be able to recall this "crucial" information when you finally encounter an item that requires it. In a sense, you are priming the pump and taking control of the situation. No rush, no panic . . . just a methodical and deliberate process of settling in before tackling the first item.

One strategy that you may have used to advantage during class exams that **is not** advisable during Step 1 is answering items out of numerical order. The strategy involves answering items you are sure of first, then items you can probably figure out with a little thought, then answering the items that are mostly blind guesses last.

Answering items in groups based on your likelihood of answering correctly makes sense on short exams with more ample time allowances. You should not use this approach on Step 1 because of the risk of mismarking answers on the scannable answer sheets. Imagine how you would feel if you realized with only a few minutes to go that you were marking out of sync on the answer sheet. Since no extra time would be allowed for you to erase and re-mark, you would lose many points and deal your confidence a terrible blow for the remainder of the exam. It's just not worth the risk.

One exception to the general rule of answering the items in numerical order is the extended matching items. Most students with whom I have talked have said that they found these items to be quicker and easier than other formats. While the list of answer choices is longer, they report that for most questions, it is quickly obvious which four or five choices fit that particular question. They also said that it was important to read the question first in order to generate a possible answer **before** scanning the list. Based on these reported experiences, you might consider answering the group of extended matching items first and then return to work the others in numerical order. To skip around more than this entails too much risk of mismarking the scannable answer sheet.

N Stands for Notations

While you are reviewing and practicing with questions, form a habit of marking key elements within test questions and using margin space to sketch little diagrams, formulas, portions of pathways, or other mnemonic aids to help you think through specific questions. By managing the information on paper, you will be freeing your mind to deal with the question more effectively because you won't have to mentally juggle all of it in your head and run the risk of forgetting a key element or making a silly calculation error. "Thinking with a pencil" also aids recall. For most students, sketching their own diagram of a mechanism brings back more of the associated details than thinking of the mechanism in their heads alone. Drawing a simplified membrane with arrows to keep track of fluid movement is more helpful than trying to recall reviewed notes on the topic. Don't handicap your recall process by forcing your mind to deal with all the information without any visual aids.

The second habit to form with regard to notations is that of marking the item itself. Key qualifying words should be circled or otherwise highlighted, such as **always**, **not**, and **except**. If the item provides detailed clinical patient data, you may want to bracket or circle any abnormal findings or significant data so they will be easy to refer to once you are dealing with the actual question being asked. Many students find it helpful to read the items that refer to the case history **first**, then read the patient data with a specific question in mind.

Reading the items that share a data set first can be particularly helpful in the longer case history question sets. Many students have reported feeling frustrated after they had laboriously worked through a case history filled with abnormal findings and lab data, all the while trying to determine the diagnosis. Reaching the final lines of the case history, they discovered that the diagnosis was given and the item asked about a related aspect such as the drug most typically given to treat the disorder or some aspect of the physiology that was disrupted by that disease. They had wasted valuable time trying to reach a diagnosis because that was what they expected to be asked.

As you examine possible responses to a particular item, form a consistent habit of noting those that you have eliminated, perhaps by putting a slash through the corresponding letter. Denote remaining choices with a "T" or a "?." Use available white space to jot down graphs or do calculations. "Thinking with a pencil" helps you concentrate, avoid careless errors, and manage the information in the items more efficiently. Diagrams and other visual aids increase your chances of recalling information.

I Stands for Ignoring

During almost any standardized examination, you will have to train yourself to ignore a number of distractions. In fact, you can begin this process of training during your review process by occasionally studying in a more public place such as the school library or cafeteria. If you are easily distracted or find your mind wandering, deal with the problem directly. Don't simply expect the tendency to solve itself. Try keeping a small card next to review materials and putting a tally mark on the card each time you notice that your concentration has wandered. The very act of tallying can decrease the frequency. As you see the marks adding up, it normally serves to make your motivation to concentrate stronger. It is a crude sort of behavior modification training and it often is quite effective!

During the actual exam, there will most likely be proctors circulating or calling out time intervals. Someone near you may jiggle a leg or tap a pencil. If you allow these noises to break into your train of thought, you will not be using time effectively and your anxiety or frustration levels may interfere with doing your best. The chief way to lessen the chance for distraction during the exam is to prepare beforehand by learning to ignore external movement or sounds by dealing with them during your reviewing. A few students I have talked with actually purchased ear plugs to wear during Step 1, but they used them before as well to get used to them. Others coped with the problem by spending a few hours each day reviewing in a cafe or other area with a lot of traffic and background noise. If you can concentrate in a cafeteria, you will have less trouble doing so in a relatively quiet examination room.

Internal distractions are just as much a problem for many students. Anxious thoughts about how you are doing, allowing yourself to become upset or angry with yourself about material you should have gotten to in your review but didn't, checking the clock every 5 minutes, or dwelling on a particularly difficult question you came to 20 minutes ago—all of these interrupt your thought process, sap your confidence, and tend to make you easily confused and hesitant about using what you remember to answer questions. Train yourself to have a positive attitude that says "I can handle this. I studied as well as I could and I can do fine on this exam." Many students find it helps to take some time a few weeks before the exam to sit down and make a special "talisman" card. On the card, they write a brief summary of their positive skills and character traits, something like the following:

> I am an intelligent, caring person who will make a fine doctor. I did well

on the MCAT. I studied hard and I can handle tests just fine. I'm going to hang in there, use strategies to handle tough items, and finish all the items in each booklet.

They take their cards out frequently during the final weeks and days before the exam, whenever they feel nervous or down on themselves, and read them out loud. Some practice visualizing themselves in a past experience where they performed some action very well under pressure. They try to reexperience how they felt, remembering the experience in as much detail as possible: what they wore, what the setting looked like, how they felt after they dealt with the problem so successfully.

If you practice either the "talisman" card or visualization techniques for several weeks before Step 1, you will be able to take a 30-second mental break from the test if needed to calm yourself and shed negative thoughts and feelings, and then return to the task with a renewed sense of calm confidence. Like preparing to compete in an athletic event, preparing to do well on a long, 2-day examination involves psychological preparation as much as it does reviewing content material. You must train to perform well on all fronts—cognitively, psychologically, and physically. If you do, there will be fewer points lost due to forgetting, self-defeating thoughts, and fatigue. Aim for the Greek ideal of a sound mind in a sound body and you won't be disappointed in the results.

C Stands for Checking

This is the last step in our no-PANIC approach to taking tests. As you recall from our discussion on pacing earlier, you aren't going to go back over items in most cases. Therefore, the checking referred to here deals with what you should do just before you color in the bubble on the scannable answer sheet. Once again, any patterns you discovered in analyzing your errors on the Diagnostic Pretest should be considered first. Do you routinely lose points by changing answers from right to wrong? Then remember the rule that you will only change an answer if you check the stem of the question and find that you actually misread the question.

Checking back over the information given in a question before recording your answer can help you eliminate most careless errors. Did you calculate correctly? Is the size of your numerical answer reasonable, given the information in the question? Do the units agree with what you should expect? Are you about to enter your response in the bubble that corresponds to the item number? Pay special attention to any questions of the type that you tend to miss, such as negatively phrased questions or very long items with a lot of information. Did you ignore a crucial bit of information about a patient with a long case history? All of these are common sources of careless errors, made without the test taker even being aware that the item was answered incorrectly. He felt confident about his own thought process as he answered the item and never realized that, in a sense, he just answered a question that wasn't being asked.

If you have time, quickly check over the answer sheet(s), scanning for double marks, incomplete erasures, or blanks. Check to make sure that all identifying information including your Step 1 identification number has been filled in. Step 1 is no place to "shoot yourself in the foot" by making errors you could easily have caught by checking.

Practicing Strategic Test Taking

Now that you have planned a rational approach to reviewing the basic science material you need for Step 1 and have seen how analyzing your error patterns can help you learn to avoid the type of mistakes to which you are most prone when answering multiple-choice questions, you should be ready to put these skills to practice. This section utilizes many items from the Diagnostic Pretest to model the use of specific test-taking strategies. To gain the most from this section of the book, it will be helpful if you try to recreate your own thinking about the repeated items before reading the item discussions. Then you will be able to see clearly which approach **you** took and what alternative approaches were possible to take with that item. The final chapter of this book consists of a 350-item practice test, which will give you ample opportunity to practice using the new strategies introduced here.

Once you have completed this book, continue trying the new strategies each time you work through practice questions during your review for Step 1. The more frequently you use questions and get into the habit of thinking strategically as well as drawing on your basic science knowledge base when you answer questions, the more likely it becomes that you will maximize your performance when you actually take the Step 1 examination. As with any new skill, it takes lots of hands-on practice time for a technique to become internalized or to reach the stage where doing it is automatic. This is what you should be aiming for during your preparation period.

One point that should be made clear at the start is that the group of strategies you will learn to use do not apply to every single multiple-choice question you will ever encounter. As one example, item 1 in the Diagnostic Pretest deals with a respiratory physiology problem. Given data from a patient's pulmonary function testing, you are asked to determine which set of values is consistent with a diagnosis of pulmonary fibrosis.

1. A 32-year-old office worker, complaining of shortness of breath, had pulmonary function testing that resulted in a diagnosis of pulmonary fibrosis. Which of the sets of values below is consistent with the diagnosis?
   A. FEV_1/FVC = 82%, IC = 3.4 L, FRC = 2.80 L, and TV = 500 ml
   B. FVC = 3.2 L, FEV_1 = 2.00 L, TLC = 6.20 L, and RV = 3.00 L
   C. FEV_1/FVC = 54%, FRC = 4.80 L, and RV = 2.30 L
   D. FVC = 2.00 L, FEV_1 = 1.80 L, TLC = 3.00 L, and RV = 1.00 L
   E. None of these value sets is consistent with the diagnosis.

With some recall of the physiologic principles related to this topic, you might be able to reason that pulmonary fibrosis is an interstitial lung disorder, and therefore you would select an answer choice with a reduced total lung capacity (TLC). Choice D, since it offers the lowest TLC value, is the answer most likely to be correct. Without this specific recall about pulmonary fibrosis, however, you would have no reasoning to apply. This example also illustrates the close interconnection between strategy use and knowledge base. The more you recall about a topic, the more likely it is that you will be able to employ reasoning strategies as well. Let's examine item 2 next.

2. Which of the following serves as a precursor for testosterone?
   A. estrone

B. cholesterol
C. aldosterone
D. cortisol
E. estriol

Assuming that you could not recall the synthetic pathways for each of these substances and thus identify the precursor directly, a useful approach would be to look at the group of answer choices and use what you could recall about each to aid your reasoning. Choice B, cholesterol, is the only substance that is a dietary component, and therefore readily available to serve as raw material for a synthetic process. Several of the others were final products themselves, which would make them unlikely candidates to be precursors in the synthesis of testosterone. Thus, it would make sense to select B as your answer.

Item 3 lends itself to reasoning to an even greater degree.

3. Conduction velocity along a myelinated nerve fiber is
   A. directly proportional to fiber diameter
   B. directly proportional to extracellular resistance
   C. inversely proportional to the thickness of the myelin coat
   D. directly proportional to the extent of demyelination
   E. inversely proportional to temperature

Let's start by looking at choice B, which states that if extracellular resistance goes up, velocity will also increase. That's not very logical since increased resistance is normally going to slow something down. Choice C is problematic. Since one function of the myelin coat is to speed things up, it doesn't seem likely that speed would decrease as the myelin coat got thicker. I would put this choice on hold and move on. Choice D almost says the opposite of choice C in that it claims that the less myelination, the faster the velocity; since this is false, rule D out. Choice E relates nerve conduction speed to temperature. It seems logical that if temperature affects conduction, it would be a direct relationship in that the colder (lower temperature) the nerve, the more slowly it would conduct, which is a possible reason why icing an injury dulls the pain. Therefore, we could rule out E as well. Now let's look at choice A. If a nerve were like a highway, it might well be that the wider it was, the faster traffic could move. Since there is no obvious reason to suppose that width might not be related to speed, this would be the best reasoned guess for this item. It turns out that choice A is the correct answer.

Look carefully at item 4 for an example of a different sort.

4. Which of the following sequences of enzyme activities is required for excision/repair of DNA?
   A. endonuclease, exonuclease, polymerase, ligase
   B. exonuclease, endonuclease, polymerase, ligase
   C. exonuclease, polymerase, endonuclease, ligase
   D. polymerase, exonuclease, endonuclease, ligase
   E. exonuclease, ligase, polymerase, endonuclease

Notice that this question deals with the proper sequence of events in a mechanism or process. With items like this, there are few reasoning strategies to apply. The choices are also quite likely to be very balanced, that is, the specific stages are represented in nearly all choices, with only their sequence varying from one choice to the next. As a consequence, the only way to increase the odds of making a correct choice is to know details of the mechanism or process itself. For example, in this item, if you knew that the repair process for DNA begins with an endonuclease, you would already have the correct answer. If you only knew that the final step in repairing DNA involves ligase, you would be left with four choices from which to guess (choice A is correct). As you can see, studying mechanisms and processes during your review is especially important. Not only do these dynamic aspects of human biology have powerful explanatory power, but they also lend themselves to questions about ordering that you are seldom going to be able to "figure out" without very specific recall.

Item 5 represents a typical Step 1 question that requires a mathematical calculation.

5. The length of hospitalization for eight patients who underwent a new procedure for the treatment of acute gout exacerbations was 10, 8, 7, 7, 4, 9, 9, and 6 days. The mean length of stay for this group of patients is
   A. 8.1 days
   B. 7.8 days
   C. 7.2 days
   D. 7.5 days
   E. 7.1 days

As you can see in this example, you won't need a calculator on Step 1 because the calculations are deliberately designed to be straightforward. Yet while the math is designed to be simple, it is a mistake to do the calculations in your head and not use pencil and available white space on the test booklet to work out the problem. All too often, mental calculations slip a decimal point or forget to carry a number. When this occurs, either the answer you come up with is not among the choices offered and you must waste time redoing the calculations or, worse yet, it **is** offered and you select it as the correct response without ever realizing your error.

Item 5 is easy because all you actually need to know in order to get the correct response is that the "mean" is the average. The numbers sum to 60. If you divide 60 by 8 (for the eight patients), you arrive at the correct answer, which is 7.5 days. The only other feature you should take notice of in this first example of a mathematical question is that the correct answer is one of the three middle values among the choices offered; 8.1 and 7.1 are the extreme answers. If you encounter an item that requires use of a formula that you can't recall or some other figure that you are unable to calculate for whatever reason, guess from among the three middle values offered in the answer choices and you will have a better statistical chance of guessing correctly. The reason for this is that most test writers begin by putting down the correct answer, then they vary it by moving the decimal point or by creating answers somewhat higher or lower than the correct value. You are simply reversing this by selecting from among the middle values, which are somewhat more likely to contain the original, and correct, answer.

We are not going to be looking at all of the items in the Diagnostic Pretest for two reasons. The first is that not every item lends itself to test-taking strategies and the other reason is that you need to focus your attention on the items that **do** lend themselves to strategies so that you will be able to identify when an item is worth the investment of reasoning time and when it is not. You can't afford to waste valuable testing time trying to wrestle with a question that is of the "You either know it or you don't" variety, henceforth referred to by the acronym YEKIOYD. Here are a few examples of items that require mainly rote memory so that you can see the characteristics of a YEKIOYD.

16. Abdominal tumors in newborns are most commonly due to which of the following conditions?
    A. hepatomegaly
    B. hydronephrosis
    C. mesenteric cysts
    D. ovarian tumors
    E. splenomegaly

Unless you can recall that "hydronephrosis" is the correct answer, the only strategy applicable to this item is to pick from the two choices that begin with the letter "h" since the correct response **may** have been one of these and the test writer was trying to hide it by including another condition beginning with the same letter to confuse you. That is an extremely low payoff strategy but, if you have nothing else to work with, it makes sense to invoke it because you have nothing to lose.

Here is another YEKIOYD example.

Items 118–121

Match each drug or drug category to the appropriate property.

A. Blocks dopamine receptors.
B. Can act as hypnotic agent(s).
C. Low therapeutic index.
D. Mechanism of action is unknown.
E. Block(s) reuptake of amine neurotransmitters.

118. tricyclic antidepressants
119. phenothiazines
120. benzodiazepines
121. lithium

The YEKIOYD item or item cluster, as shown above, is found more frequently in certain subject areas than in others. Microbiology, pharmacology, and biochemistry seem to lend themselves to this type of question. Perhaps it is because one must simply memorize a certain number of bug, drug, or enzyme names in order to link them in family groupings that, in turn, give you a way to organize their associated features or effects. Whatever the reason, you can expect to see a fair number of YEKIOYDs on Step 1, although far fewer than you would have 10 years ago. A serious effort has been made to write Step 1 from a more clinical perspective. This is why the exam was shortened from more than 1000 items to 800 and why so many items are now put into a clinical setting or vignette that requires the test taker to select the important data and to apply basic science principles to a patient care situation. While this change in Step 1 is a very positive development, some test takers might actually do worse on some of the clinically embedded items. Here is an example to illustrate the problem. For this item, the behavior must be matched with its appropriate defense mechanism.

44. A young man, not athletically talented but with many close friends on college teams, decides to open a sports equipment and memorabilia store next door to the college sports arena.
    A. introjection
    B. projection
    C. sublimation
    D. reaction formation
    E. denial

This question really deals with the precise meaning of psychiatric terms; it is a basic "definition" question. By placing the test taker in the position of matching a very brief vignette to the proper term for the depicted behavior, there is room for ambiguity. More than simply having to match the textbook definition to the term, a test taker must now be able to correctly interpret the vignette and **judge its meaning as the test author intended** in order to select the correct response. Experience in dealing with these clinical or situationally embedded items helps. Often, experienced test takers will reduce the prose description of a patient being wheeled into the emergency room with a certain type of injury that leads to numbness in a certain body area to its anatomical essence. Such a test taker would read the vignette and then paraphrase the stem to "so what's being asked is which nerve innervates this portion of the foot." By simplifying the question, there is less chance of making an error.

For item 44 (above), the description might be paraphrased in the test taker's mind in the following way: "This guy who can't be a jock gets some glory by associating his business and its location with athletic stardom, which is **sublimation**." You can see how slippery these items can be since a different interpretation of the same vignette might be paraphrased as "a guy who refuses to admit that he is not athletically talented and denies the truth by associating every aspect of his life with athletic success, which is **denial**." By placing a different interpretation on the same data, the defined behavior is changed as well. Your only defense against making the wrong interpretation of vignettes such as these is to avoid bringing any assumptions to the vignette that might change the perceived meaning. In the second scenario, the test taker is assuming that the young man has repeatedly denied that he is untalented athletically. The vignette simply states that he is not talented but doesn't suggest anything about how the young man depicts himself to others. Therefore, the assumption is unjustified.

Guarding against hidden assumptions can be difficult. You might try rereading the vignette with the conscious intention to check the evidence for or against the interpretation you have formed. Sometimes, reducing a clinical vignette to its basic science essence is helpful in that it changes a long complex-sounding stem describing "a young woman who was seen in a family physician's office who had a certain medical and social history, and who now presents with the following symptoms, and was found to have thus and such signs on physical examination" into a simple factual question such as "Damage to which nerve causes lid lag?"

Let's turn back to items in the Diagnostic Pretest to see other strategies that you can use on multiple-choice items.

9. Which of the following has the **lowest** metabolic clearance rate?
    A. hormone A with a half-life of 1 hour, 95% plasma binding
    B. hormone B with a half-life of 1 minute, 5% plasma binding

C. hormone C with a half-life of 1 hour, 60% plasma binding
D. hormone D with a half-life of 1 day, 99% plasma binding
E. hormone E with a half-life of 1 minute, 0.5% plasma binding

If you understand the concept of half-life, you know that the longer the half-life, the more of a substance is left after a given length of time. Also, you might recall that if something is bound to plasma, it is less easily excreted. Putting these two concepts together, you already know that you are looking for an answer choice that has a long half-life and a relatively high binding percentage. Since choice D fits both criteria, hormone D would have the lowest clearance rate. This is pure logic but its use is inextricably linked to basic definitions of half-life and binding. Again, you can see that strategies used in test taking are closely intertwined with one's knowledge of the content material.

22. A 35-year-old female patient's eyes move normally except that her left eye cannot adduct. You suspect that her CNS lesion involves the
    A. IV nucleus on the left side
    B. VI nucleus on the right side
    C. medulla
    D. left medial longitudinal fasciculus
    E. right cerebellum

In item 22, we know from the patient's data that her only abnormality is an inability to adduct the left eye. This is a very specific symptom. Now look at the choices offered. Choices C and E involve two very general brain areas, the medulla and the right cerebellum. These choices are probably too generalized in function to fit her very specific symptom. The remaining choices specify a location on either the right (choice B) or the left side (A and D). Since the test author may have been trying to mimic some facet of the correct answer in an incorrect choice, it would be better to select a left-sided answer, which would mean selecting either choice A or D. The correct response is D, which means that there would have been at least a 50% probability of getting a correct answer. Notice that several tactics were employed here: using a general science concept that specific functions are often controlled from specific areas in the brain, and that test writers frequently reuse parts of the correct response when they create incorrect answer choices.

Format cues can also help you analyze test items. For example, in a negatively phrased item that has the general form "all of the following are true about a topic **except**," you should try to step back from the choices and view them from more than one angle or perspective to determine if some common feature links four of them and leaves one standing alone. Students I have worked with have dubbed this the "Sesame Street" strategy after the little song on the children's television show that asks "Which of these things is not like the others?" Another helpful strategy for negatively stated items is to scan the choices to see if, in some sense, two of the choices are opposites of each other, as in the following example:

53. All of the following typify IgA nephropathy (Berger's disease) **except**
    A. it may result from injury of the intestinal mucosa by lectin-like molecules from wheat

B. it may be associated with alcohol abuse
C. deposits of IgA, IgG, and C3 are found in the mesangium
D. it frequently progresses to end-stage renal disease
E. its course is generally considered to be benign

Notice that choices D and E cannot both be correct since one states that this is usually a fatal disease while the other says that it isn't normally fatal. Logically, if both cannot be correct, one statement **is** the correct answer because in this format you are to identify the **incorrect** statement. (The correct answer is E.)

Here is an item demonstrating that similarity among choices in a negatively phrased item can help to rule in or rule out related choices as a group.

61. By definition, a "carcinoma" is described by all of the following **except**
   A. epithelial in origin
   B. gland-forming
   C. malignant
   D. neoplastic
   E. a subtype of cancer

Did you spot the overlapped meaning in choices C, D, and E? You can rule out all three and concentrate on choices A or B as possibly the **incorrect** statement about carcinomas. (The correct response is B.) If you could have recalled any specific examples of carcinomas and knew that the ones you remembered either were or were not gland-forming, you would have been able to answer the item correctly based on that partial recall in combination with the format cues you had already employed to narrow the choice to A or B. Perhaps you see more clearly now how strategies work synergistically with your knowledge base.

Another example illustrates how you can use cues from the format of an item to help select a correct answer.

71. Long-term regulation of arterial blood pressure
   A. is independent of carotid sinus reflexes
   B. is affected by the renin-angiotensin system
   C. depends on renal excretory function
   D. is markedly affected by changes in salt and water balance
   E. is regulated by all of the above factors

It is fairly obvious that choice D is true in that almost everyone is aware of the link between salt consumption, water retention, and high blood pressure (use of common knowledge!). Since one of the main functions of the kidney is to excrete filtered fluid wastes, which is the gist of choice D, this would also be tied to water balance and hence to blood pressure, and, thus, statement C is also true. At this point, you would automatically select E because you have identified two correct choices and therefore all must be correct given the format of the item.

Here is an item in which you can take advantage of the fact that some things are given functionally descriptive names, which is using word structure strategically.

49. Ovarian cells that transform into the corpus luteum must have receptors for

A. epidermal growth factor
B. follicle-stimulating hormone
C. inhibin
D. lutenizing hormone
E. progesterone

If the question is focusing on the factor that triggers a transformation of the ovarian cells, you would not select choice C, as inhibin is probably an inhibiting factor. Since epidermis (choice A) is associated with outer surfaces, it may not stimulate ovarian cells to transform, and I would therefore rule it out as well. Looking at the remaining choices, B, D, or E, it strikes a careful reader that a **lut**einizing hormone might be involved in the formation of the corpus **lut**eum, and, thus, I would select this as the most likely answer. While such convenient links between terms or parts of terms in the stem of the item and a specific choice don't occur with great frequency, it is important to make use of the meaning in the nomenclature of medicine when it seems appropriate.

Getting graph-related items correct doesn't usually require higher mathematics or an advanced degree in biophysics. However, you must have the attitude that graphs are helpful, not confusing. And you must be willing to examine the graphic relationships carefully, noting units and the relationships between variables that are being displayed in the graph, then relate these to what you know conceptually about the topic of the item. Try to train yourself to think positively about data tables and graphs. Rather than confusing you, such items can actually provide the information needed to arrive at the correct answer, and generally require less rote recall of information than other, far simpler-appearing items of the YEKIOYD variety. Try responding to graphic items by thinking of how much information they provide you to reason with instead of how complex they look at first glance.

Here is an example to illustrate that complex-looking items aren't necessarily the most difficult. They do trigger an almost instant "I give up" reaction from too many test takers, however. Try to fight this reflex response to data sets, diagrams, or other items so you will be able to use the revealed information to your benefit in answering the item correctly.

A hypothetical biosynthetic pathway is shown below. A microbial organism defective in one enzyme of this pathway is grown in a medium containing X. Large amounts of M and L are found in the organism but none of Z. Which enzyme has the mutation?
A. enzyme A
B. enzyme B
C. enzyme C
D. enzyme D
E. enzyme E

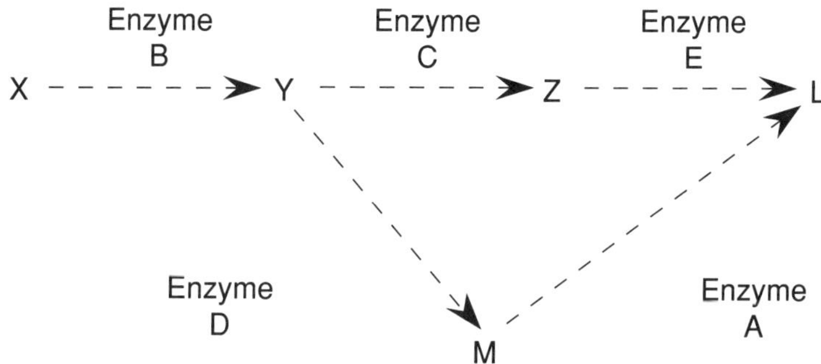

By studying the diagram and realizing that the organism is able to produce M and L but no Z, you can conclude that enzymes D, A, and B must be functional, since all three would be required to produce L. If no Z is being produced, it must be because enzyme C is defective. Why can't enzyme E be the defective one? Because enzyme E only works on substance Z as it is converted to L, if it were defective, you could still get Z but you would have to go through the X→Y→M→L pathway to produce any L. Clearly, the diagram displays the correct response. Your job is to be ready to use the information provided to see what is revealed.

Let's review the strategies that have been used in relation to items in this section.

Reasoning with Recalled Information or with Information Given in the Item

This is probably the most powerful of all test-taking strategies because it allows you to use logic to extend what you know to the particular situation being depicted in a question. Reasoning subsumes or carries within it other, lesser strategies such as use of word parts and format cues to rule in or rule out specific answer choices. In the actual practice of medicine, especially in the area of diagnosis or determining which test should be performed, physicians make daily use of reasoning and logic to determine diagnostic probabilities and to decide which tests are appropriate and in what order. Probabilistic reasoning is used almost unconsciously when physicians form hypotheses about what diseases may be producing observed symptoms and signs, as more common diseases are considered first and rarer conditions are suspected only when common ones have been ruled out. Reason is a powerful tool in real life and it is also a powerful tool in test taking.

Using All the Information Given in a Question

Test takers have a tendency to forget a crucial piece of data when they are thinking through long items that are densely packed with information. To avoid forgetting a key fact and therefore failing to test possible answers against **all** the given information, get into the habit of marking up the item by highlighting techniques, such as circling abnormal findings, underlining important qualifiers, or crossing through irrelevant data. This helps you manage "information overload" and keeps you focused on the most important elements in judging possible choices. It also saves time if you find that you need to return to a long stem or clinical vignette as the key data are already identified.

Using Word Structure and Word Nuances

If you are a native speaker of English, you have an advantage in that you can read for subtleties in the language used in items. This ability especially pays off in definition items and, in combination with reasoning and logic, when word parts are shared between key words in the item stem and certain answer choices. If you think physicians don't employ this skill in dealing with patients, ask one to talk about the many descriptions of pain that patients have used to convey their symptoms or the verbal hints that patients provide through their word choices about psychosocial factors or the severity of their conditions. Like any other clue, however, it isn't revealing if you don't notice it is there.

Format Cues and the Sesame Street Principle

With the changes in the testing format on the Step 1 exam, there are two main item types in which format can be helpful in selecting answers that are more likely to be correct. The format that lends itself most frequently to this approach is the negatively phrased item. It is extremely helpful to step back from the choices in a negatively phrased item to see if they have some common factor. If four choices seem similar or overlap in some basic respect, the remaining choice is usually the correct response. This is the basis of the Sesame Street principle. If you can determine that even two or three of the choices are similar, you have ruled out this group and can then guess from the remaining (fewer) choices, which increases the odds of responding correctly.

On occasion, you will encounter a positively stated item that has an "all of the above are correct" choice. With this type of item, determining that even two statements are correct automatically determines that "all" is the correct response.

Analyzing Diagrams, Data Sets, and Graphs

Even if mathematics is not your forte, you can learn to study the information that is provided in these items to look for patterns or draw logical conclusions about a topic. Often, everything you need to answer the item correctly is displayed, but you must have the will to seek it and work with the information. Skipping over the graph with the hope that you can answer an item based on the prose stem and answer choices offered is usually as fruitful as picking an answer at random. With graphic or diagrammed information, you have to be willing to examine the data carefully and then, with a minimal amount of calculation or reasoning, you will frequently arrive at the correct answer. Remember, the more information that is provided with the item, the less memorized knowledge you have to provide to determine the correct answer.

Using General Knowledge and Experience

Realize that you have a great deal of information about the world besides that which you learned in basic science lecture halls over the past few years. When the correct answer isn't obvious, don't be afraid to use common sense, science information, or epidemiology data revealed in the media to aid your reasoning. Reasoning with extreme or prototypical examples from real life is an invaluable adjunct to what you have studied in medical school. As one of my students expressed it, "Don't take tests wearing horse blinders."

Sorting Choices into Groups

As you saw in a number of examples discussed in this section, choices often fall into groupings, for example, two very specific choices and three more general choices, or two choices that deal with restrictive lung diseases and three that are obstructive lung diseases. Use these groupings to rule groups of choices in or out as you reason through an item. If you approach an item with the assumption that all choices are independent possibilities, you will waste time by evaluating each choice independently. Seeing the grouping among choices also helps put the item into a clearer context, relating the item to groups of entities as you learned them in class. Matching a patient's symptoms to known disease presentations is pattern recognition applied to the clinical setting. Pattern recognition is just as helpful in becoming an effective test taker.

These are the power strategies of a skilled test taker. There are several other strategies that have a lower payoff; that is, they are less likely to lead to selecting a correct answer. If you encounter an item for which you have no useful recall, however, the lesser strategies are worth using because the odds of getting the item correct are already 1 in 5. Here is a quick summary of these "best guess" and lower power strategies.

Select from Choices That Share Terms

This strategy is based on the principle that the test author has reused elements of the correct response in the incorrect choices that he or she creates in order to try to "hide" the correct answer or just because this is an easy way of creating wrong responses.

Select from the Middle Values

In items in which the answer choices can be ordered or ranked in some way, you would select a choice from the middle three choices, assuming you had no knowledge that would guide you to a particular answer. Based on the same idea as the strategy above, this strategy assumes that the test writer varied up and down from the original, correct response to create false choices, so that the extreme values (the highest and lowest) of those offered are less likely to be correct. You should note that this strategy is only to be used when you do not have the knowledge to arrive at an answer and are forced to guess. If you calculated an answer that agreed with a value that was highest or lowest, you should choose that answer and not one of the middle values.

Using the strategies demonstrated in this section is not difficult, but it does require developing a frame of mind that seeks opportunities to use these approaches when you work through test items. If you try questions during your review for Step 1 in the "business as usual" habitual way, you will not improve in your ability to make better, more reasoned answers to test questions. The practice questions that follow are grouped by subject, so you may wish to try each set as you finish reviewing an area. You may also want to save this Posttest for later in your review process, so that you can attempt to apply all the various strategies that have been discussed. The items are quite representative of what you will see on Step 1, except that they are grouped in subject areas. Whichever way you decide to use the Posttest, remember that you need to consciously apply strategies in repeated practice sessions with test questions in order to make the strategies an automatic and comfortable part of your test-taking habits. Good luck on Step 1.

3

A Posttest with Explanations

Anatomy

1. A 32-year-old man was stricken with viral pneumonia and had an unremitting fever of over 103°F for 4 days. One result of his illness was the lack of any viable sperm upon his recovery from the illness. How long would it take for this young man to become capable of producing a viable sperm sample?
   A. 5 days
   B. 2 weeks
   C. 3 weeks
   D. 2 months
   E. 6 months

Items 2–6

The diagram below shows a human fetus in its second month of development. Match each of the labeled structures to its appropriate name.

2. amnion
3. chorion
4. umbilical cord
5. amnionic cavity
6. yolk sac

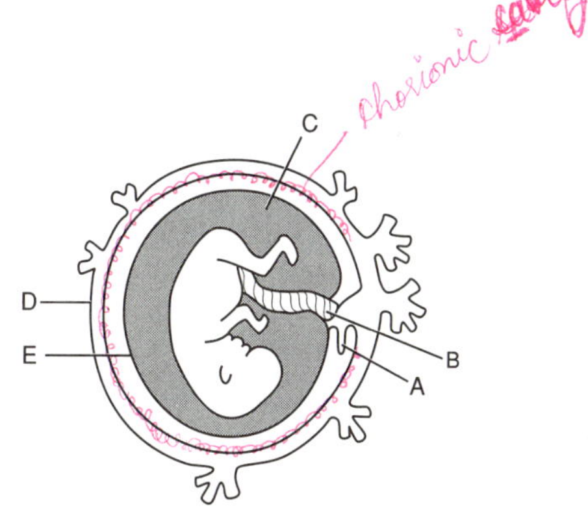

7. An 18-year-old black female is about to marry a black male. She has a younger brother who has sickle cell disease. She and her fiancé seek genetic counseling to learn the chance that any offspring might have the disease. The genetic counselor calculates the likelihood that they will have an affected child as

A. 1/15
B. 1/25
C. 1/75
D. 1/250
E. 1/300

8. In the US, warning labels are now carried on many products to lessen the likelihood that pregnant women will give birth to infants with defects. Of the substances listed below, which is known to be teratogenic with chronic use by the mother?
A. alcohol
B. coffee
C. heroin
D. marijuana
E. nicotine

9. At the present time, the most frequently used mode of treatment for genetic diseases is
A. treating symptoms of the disease
B. treating metabolic abnormalities
C. transplanting organs
D. gene therapy
E. palliative care

10. You are asked to assume responsibilities for your retiring partner. In examining one of his patients, who suffers from Turner's syndrome, you would expect all of the following to be noted in this patient **except**
A. a lack of follicular development
B. a streak ovary
C. a uterus
D. a webbed neck
E. menses

11. The production and maintenance of all the components of connective tissue extracellular matrix are the task of the
A. fibroblast
B. lymphocyte
C. macrophage
D. mast cell
E. mesothelial cell

12. You are treating a young female patient who has undergone a prolonged period of starvation. Fat from which of the following body stores would be the **last** to be utilized?
A. mesenteric fat
B. retroperitoneal fat
C. subcutaneous fat of the breasts
D. pads of the hands and feet
E. subcutaneous fat of the anterior thighs

13. A 12-year-old boy suffers injury to nerves in the left arm. All of the

following changes might be observed following the damage to the axons in his arm **except**

A. chromatolysis in the soma
B. degeneration of the axon up to several internodes from the injury site
C. movement of the axonal nucleus to an eccentric position
D. neuritic outgrowth from the stump
E. total degeneration of the myelin sheath back to the initial segment

14. An erythrocyte in circulation typically survives about
    A. 2 weeks
    B. 6 weeks
    C. 2 months
    D. 4 months
    E. 6 months

15. A 40-year-old construction worker is seriously injured in an accident. Due to hemorrhaging caused by his injuries, which of the following might be stimulated to begin producing erythrocytes?
    A. kidneys, liver, and spleen
    B. kidneys, yellow marrow, and spleen
    C. kidneys, thymus, and lymph nodes
    D. lymph nodes, spleen, and thymus
    E. yellow marrow, spleen, and liver

16. Inhalation is a complex, coordinated event. Identify the **incorrect** statement among the following statements describing what takes place during inhalation.
    A. Elastic fibers in alveolar septa contract.
    B. Some intercostal muscles contract.
    C. The diaphragm contracts.
    D. The bronchi and bronchiole lumens become wider.
    E. A partial vacuum is created in the thoracic cavity.

17. In a patient with a severed inferior laryngeal nerve, the innervation of which of the following muscles would be intact?
    A. cricothyroid
    B. lateral cricoarytenoid
    C. posterior cricoarytenoid
    D. transverse arytenoid
    E. thyroarytenoid

18. A 13-year-old hockey player is brought into the ER with a suspected carpal fracture. Which of the following bones is usually involved in this type of injury?
    A. the capitate
    B. the hamate
    C. the lunate
    D. the pisiform
    E. the scaphoid

19. You are performing the cardiovascular portion of a physical examination on a 28-year-old man. You place the stethoscope over the apex, in the left fifth intercostal space. This is the best position for you to hear the sounds of the
    A. aortic valve
    B. pulmonary artery
    C. mitral valve
    D. tricuspid valve
    E. apex of the heartbeat

20. While examining the back of a 17-year-old female patient, you notice a lateral curvature of the vertebral column. The term you would use to denote this abnormality is
    A. a "gorilla" rib
    B. a ruptured disk
    C. kyphosis
    D. lordosis
    E. scoliosis

21. Injury to which of the following nerves would result in a "claw" hand?
    A. axillary
    B. median
    C. musculocutaneous
    D. radial
    E. ulnar

22. You are attending a sporting event when an 8-year-old boy sitting in the row behind you begins choking. His mother states that he had been eating a small piece of candy. As you perform a Heimlich maneuver, you speculate that the candy, if inhaled, most likely became lodged in the child's
    A. larynx
    B. left bronchus
    C. right bronchus
    D. trachea
    E. None of these is likely.

23. A 13-year-old female patient recently suffered facial injuries in a car accident and now complains that she has no sensation in the skin of her left cheek. You suspect that she may have damage in which of the following nerves?
    A. the auriculotemporal
    B. the buccal branch of the trigeminal
    C. the mental
    D. the zygomaticofacial
    E. the zygomaticotemporal

24. You are dreaming that you have been miniaturized and injected into a living human. As you journey through the heart, you observe an oval, depressed, thinned-out area in the medial wall of the left atrium. This structure is called the

A. valvula foraminis ovalis
B. fossa ovalis
C. opening of the coronary sinus
D. septomarginal trabecula
E. terminal crest

Items 25–29

Match the cell bodies and neuron types listed below to their proper neuroanatomic locations.

A. first-order neuron cell bodies
B. third-order sensory neurons
C. sensory, motor, and association neurons
D. postganglionic sympathetic motor cells
E. no first-order sensory neurons

25. thalamus
26. sensory ganglia of cranial nerves
27. dorsal root ganglia of spinal nerves
28. cortex
29. cerebellum

Items 30–35

The diagram below shows the spinal cord at the midcervical level. Match the labeled sections to the appropriate terms.

30. anterior corticospinal tract
31. lateral corticospinal tract
32. lateral spinothalamic tract
33. fasciculus cuneatus
34. rubrospinal tract
35. anterior spinocerebellar tract

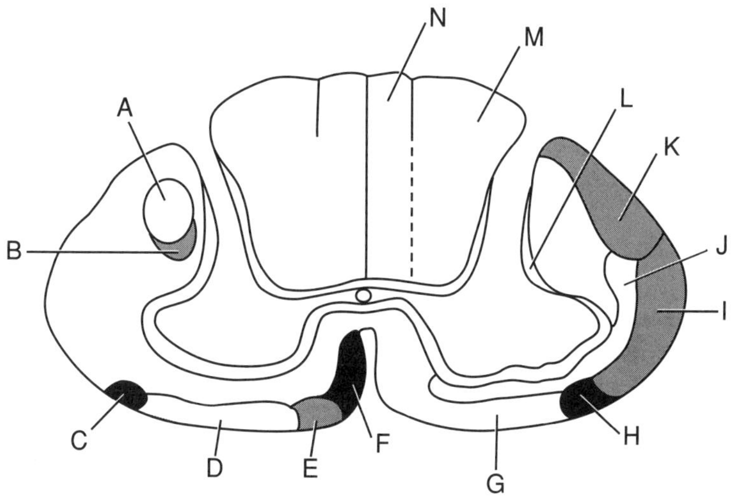

Items 36–39

Match each description to the appropriate term.

A. Forms the 13 protofilaments in microtubules.
B. Present in flagella, has ATPase activity.
C. A type of intermediate filament.
D. Present in epithelial tonofilaments.
E. A globular protein present in thin filaments of muscle cells.

36. desmin
37. tubulin
38. actin
39. dynein

40. Identify the **incorrect** statement regarding the nucleolus.
    A. Contains strands of DNA.
    B. Can recover from ultraviolet radiation.
    C. Contains the genes for RNA synthesis.
    D. Contains ribosome precursors.
    E. Contains the nucleolar organizer region.

41. All of the following statements correctly describe basement membranes **except**
    A. Present in lymphatic capillaries.
    B. Fine structure varies greatly with location and function.
    C. Contain highly glycosylated type IV collagen.
    D. May adhere to epithelial cells via hemidesmosomes.
    E. Function as a selective barrier in the glomerulus.

Items 42–45

Match the type of bone to the appropriate description.

A. compact bone
B. spongy bone
C. both
D. neither

42. Has a rich blood supply.
43. Found in the metaphysis of long bones.
44. Contains few osteocytes.
45. Major component in the shaft of long bones.

46. Each of the following statements about cardiac muscle tissue is correct **except**
    A. its cells are joined by intercalated disks
    B. it contains abundant gap junctions
    C. it is found in proximal sections of the aorta and vena cava
    D. it contains many sarcomeres
    E. its satellite cells facilitate hypertrophy

Items 47–50

Match the descriptions below to the appropriate enteroendocrine cells.

A. A cells
B. D cells
C. EC cells
D. G cells
E. I cells
F. K cells
G. L cells
H. S cells

47. Present in the colon and small intestine, they secrete glucagon.
48. They secrete serotonin and are scattered throughout the gastric mucosa.
49. Present in the duodenum and pylorus, they secrete gastrin.
50. They are present only in the upper one third of the gastric mucosa.

51. Which of the following statements regarding the seminal vesicles is **false**?
    A. They are paired diverticula of the ductus deferens.
    B. They are true glands.
    C. They lie superior to the prostate gland.
    D. They are lined with pseudostratified epithelium.
    E. They contain abundant smooth muscle.

Explanations for Anatomy Items

1. D

2. E, 3. D, 4. B, 5. C, 6. A (Moore 1988, 104–109). The outermost fetal membrane, the chorion, is separated from the inner membrane, the amnion, by a small space called the chorionic cavity. It is within this space that the yolk sac, another fetal membrane, attaches to the umbilical cord. The developing human lies within the amnion, in the amniotic cavity, attached to the placenta by the umbilical cord and surrounded by amniotic fluid.

7. C

8. A (Moore 1988, 146–147). Fetal alcohol syndrome results from chronic alcohol use during pregnancy. Infants born to alcoholic mothers present with intrauterine growth retardation, mental retardation, abnormal facial features, abnormal palmar creases, and congenital heart disease. "Maternal alcohol abuse is thought to be the most common cause of mental retardation."

9. A

10. E (Moore 1988, 132–138). Turner's syndrome results from monosomy

of the X chromosome in females (XO). These patients are characterized by a webbed neck and broad chest. Although these females possess all the appropriate sexual organs, there is no sexual maturation and no menses.

11. A (Alberts et al. 1989, 803, 813–815, 986–987). The fibroblast is a multipotent cell that produces most extracellular matrix molecules, including the structural collagenous network as well as the adhesive glycoproteins. As these cells produce the matrix, they also organize it by pulling the collagen fibers into cables as they migrate. This organization makes possible the formation of ligaments and tendons.

12. D

13. E

14. D

15. D

16. A

17. A

18. E

19. C

20. E

21. E

22. C

23. B

24. B (Moore 1988, 296–300). In the embryonic heart, blood may pass from the right atrium into the left atrium via the foramen ovalis, an aperture in the interatrial septum. At birth, this opening closes and seals, leaving a thin-walled remnant called the fossa ovalis.

25. B

26. A

27. A

28. C

29. E

30. F

31. A

32. J

33. M

34. B

35. I

36. C, desmin (Alberts et al. 1989, 661–664). Intermediate filaments are cytoskeletal components ranging between 8 and 10 nm in diameter. This is "intermediate" in size compared to the thick and thin filaments in cells. Different intermediate filament types are specific for certain cells. Keratin is the intermediate filament characteristic for epithelial cells, while vimentin is characteristic for mesenchymal and endothelial cells. The intermediate filament that is characteristic for both smooth and striated muscle is desmin.

37. A, tubulin (Alberts et al. 1989, 646–647). Tubulin is a globular heterodimer, composed of an α- and a β-tubulin subunit. By aligning themselves into polar cables, called protofilaments, and interacting in a side-by-side manner, a hollow cord consisting of 13 protofilaments forms. This cord is a microtubule.

38. E, actin (Alberts et al. 1989, 616–623). Actin filaments, or F actin, are composed of long chains of globular, or G, actin. Myosin, the thick filament of muscle, interacts with F actin and hydrolyzes ATP to begin the sliding action that is a muscle contraction.

39. B, dynein (Alberts et al. 1989, 648–649). The back-and-forth motion of a cilium is made possible by the molecule dynein and its interaction with microtubules. Dynein is composed of three globular heads attached to a microtubule by small filaments. The globular heads, which interact with adjacent microtubules, hydrolyze ATP, causing the head to slide along the microtubules. With all dynein molecules acting in concert, the net result is ciliary movement.

40. B (Alberts et al. 1989, 541–544). Large open loops of DNA, containing the genes for rRNA arranged into a nucleolar organized region, form the nucleolus. It is within this region that the rRNA first interacts with protein subunits to begin the formation of a ribosome. All DNA is sensitive to UV radiation.

41. A (Junqueira and Kelley 1989, 66, 227). Basement membranes are found in lymphatic capillaries. The basement membrane is a structure consisting predominantly of type IV collagen, proteoglycans, and adhesive glycoproteins that underlies epithelial layers, allowing the cells to attach via hemidesmosomes. Although the composition of basement membranes

remains relatively consistent, the organization and functions can vary dramatically. The kidneys use the basement membrane as a selective filter, while the lymphatic capillaries have relatively no basement membrane that would interfere with fluid adsorption.

42. C (Junqueira and Kelley 1989, 143–145). Both bone types are highly vascularized. In compact bone, the haversian system centers around a blood vessel. Spongy bone, a location for hematopoiesis, contains many capillaries with which to receive nutrients.

43. B (Junqueira and Kelley 1989, 143–145). Spongy bone is found in the epiphysis and metaphysis, and as a minor component lining the central shaft of long bone. Also, the diploë, or center of flat bones, is composed of spongy bone.

44. D, neither (Junqueira and Kelley 1989, 143–145). Osteocytes are bone-matrix producing cells and are abundant in compact and spongy bone.

45. A, compact bone (Junqueira and Kelley 1989, 143–145). The shaft, or diaphysis, is largely composed of an outer compact bone layer with a central marrow cavity lined with a thin layer of spongy bone.

46. E (Junqueira and Kelley 1989, 194–210). Cardiac muscle satellite cells facilitate hypertrophy. Cardiac and skeletal muscle are types of striated muscle and as such, have fibers arranged into basic elements called sarcomeres. The intercalated disk, containing many gap junctions, is a structure characteristic of cardiac muscle and allows the cells to function together as a syncitium. Satellite cells are those cells that can be stimulated to become new muscle cells in skeletal muscle. Cardiac muscle contains no satellite cells.

47. G

48. C

49. D

50. A

51. B

References

Alberts B, et al. (eds): Molecular Biology of the Cell. 2nd ed. New York: Garland, 1989.

Junqueira L, Kelley R (eds): Basic Histology. 6th ed. Norwalk, CT: Appleton & Lange, 1989.

Moore K (ed): The Developing Human. 4th ed. Philadelphia: Saunders, 1988.

Biochemistry

1. Genetic complementation tests are used to determine whether two different mutants carry mutations in the same
   A. cistron
   B. chromosome
   C. plasmid
   D. muton
   E. recon

2. A secondary mutation that eliminates the phenotypic consequence of a primary mutation is called a
   A. suppressor
   B. inducer
   C. repressor
   D. operator
   E. recombinant

3. A woman whose father had classic hemophilia, a deficiency of factor VIII (antihemophilic factor), is married to a normal man. On the average, each of the following members of her family would be expected to have, or be carriers of, hemophilia **except**
   A. half of her sons
   B. half of her paternal uncles
   C. half of her brothers
   D. half of her daughters
   E. one fourth of the sons of all her daughters

4. A population of proliferating cells has a generation time of 24 hours. The G1 phase of the cell cycle is 6 hours long. The G2 phase is 3 hours long, and cell division requires 1 hour. What is the length of the DNA synthesis period?
   A. 4 hours
   B. 9 hours
   C. 10 hours
   D. 14 hours
   E. 18 hours

5. A 12-year-old boy presented at a dermatology clinic with a skin tumor on the right cheek. He had always avoided exposure to sunlight because it made his skin blister. His skin had scattered areas of hyperpigmentation and other areas looked mildly atrophied. If the dermatologist's tentative diagnosis of xeroderma pigmentosum is correct, which of the following would be true of this boy's condition?
   A. His condition would be inherited in an autosomal dominant pattern.
   B. The defect is in an exonuclease involved in DNA repair.
   C. Sunscreen used would have little or no effect.
   D. He has a 1000-fold greater chance of developing skin cancer than normal individuals.
   E. Enzyme therapy will help prevent future tumor development.

6. Which of the following statements regarding cystic fibrosis (CF) is **incorrect**?
   A. CF is the most common serious genetic disease among whites in North America.
   B. CF is inherited as an autosomal recessive disease.
   C. CF is a disease of the endocrine glands.
   D. Frequent infections of *Staphylococcus aureus* and *Pseudomonas aeruginosa* are typical.
   E. Pancreatic enzyme should be given with each meal.

7. The amino acid that is most likely to be located in the interior of a globular protein is
   A. alanine
   B. aspartic acid
   C. glutamic acid
   D. histidine
   E. lysine

Items 8–9

In the oxygen dissociation graph below, the three curves are lettered A, B, and C. Select the curve that most closely corresponds to each statement. Lettered choices may be used once, more than once, or not at all.

8. Blood sample taken from an individual who resides in a Himalayan village.

9. Blood sample taken from an individual with an enzymatic defect that leads to lowered levels of 2,3-diphosphoglycerate (2,3-DPG).

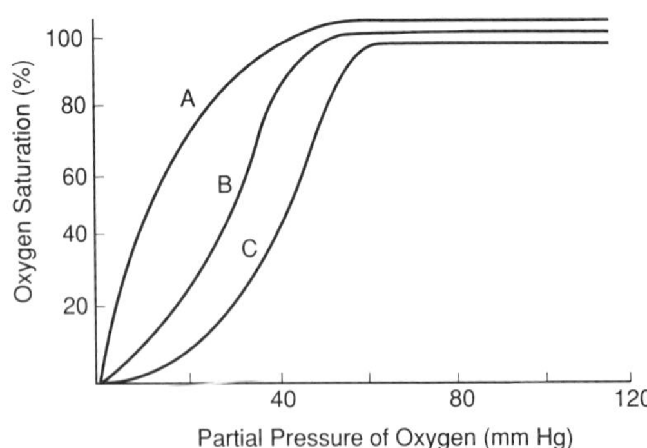

10. Enzymes catalyzing the cleavage of C-C, C-O, C-N, and other bonds by elimination reactions to yield double bonds or by adding groups to double bonds are examples of which enzyme class?
    A. oxidoreductase
    B. transferase
    C. hydrolase
    D. lyase
    E. ligase

11. Transcriptional control can modulate metabolic flux by affecting levels of which of the following proteins?
    A. acetyl CoA carboxylase
    B. HMG-CoA reductase
    C. glucose 6-phosphate dehydrogenase
    D. citrate cleavage enzyme
    E. all of the above

12. All of the following are causes of B-complex vitamin deficiency **except**
    A. failure of the liver to synthesize the vitamins
    B. lack of dietary intake
    C. intake of various drugs, including alcohol
    D. strict vegetarianism
    E. surgical removal of the stomach or intestine

13. Blood glucose levels are maintained through all of the following **except**
    A. degradation of liver glycogen
    B. gluconeogenesis from glycerol of fat in diet
    C. synthesis of glucose from lactate
    D. breakdown of body protein in a hepatectomized dog
    E. conversion of alanine to glucose

14. Identify the **false** statement regarding the Fc fragment of the IgG molecule.
    A. It is glycosylated.
    B. It can be obtained by limited proteolysis of IgG by papain.
    C. It contains only heavy chains.
    D. It forms Bence Jones protein in patients with myeloma.
    E. It mediates complement fixation in intact IgG.

15. The enzyme that is missing in patients with alcaptonuria is
    A. phenylalanine hyroxylase
    B. 4-malethylacetoacetate isomerase
    C. 4-hydroxyphenylpyruvate dioxygenase
    D. homogentisate 1,2-dioxygenase
    E. tyrosine transaminase

16. The reaction catalyzed by enterokinase (enteropeptidase) is essential for the digestion of proteins because enterokinase
    A. activates trypsinogen, the first step in activating other proteases
    B. activates pancreatic amylase
    C. activates pepsinogen
    D. activates aminooligopeptidases in jejunal brush-border membranes
    E. can directly release free amino acids from dietary proteins

17. All of the following statements about essential amino acids are correct **except**
    A. they are supplied by the diet
    B. they may be precursors of other amino acids
    C. they may be precursors of epinephrine and serotonin

D. they include lysine, tryptophan, and phenylalanine
E. they include glutamic acid, alanine, and aspartic acid

18. Which statement below most accurately describes the phenomenon of uncoupling in oxidative phosphorylation?
A. Formation of ATP continues, but oxidation of TCA cycle intermediates stops.
B. ATP formation stops but oxidation of TCA cycle intermediates continues.
C. ATP formation stops because the TCA cycle is inhibited.
D. Mitochondrial metabolism is blocked.
E. The movement of ATP-ADP across the mitochondrial inner membrane is inhibited.

19. Which of the following molecules links the urea cycle with the citric acid cycle?
A. α-ketoglutarate
B. succinyl CoA
C. pyruvate
D. citrulline
E. fumarate

20. The largest factor in protein folding and stabilization is contributed by
A. hydrogen bonds
B. coulombic interactions
C. dipole-dipole interactions
D. microenvironmental factors
E. hydrophobic interactions

21. Hemoglobin and myoglobin share all of the following characteristics **except** their
A. iron content by weight
B. oxidation state of iron
C. coordination of the iron atom
D. oxygen binding curve
E. percent α-helix content

22. In the treatment of hyperlipidemia, which of the following is most effective as a **single-dose therapy** to raise HDL, lower cholesterol, and lower triglycerides?
A. niacin
B. HMG-CoA reductase inhibitor
C. fibroic acid
D. probucol
E. bile acid–binding resin

23. In congenital adrenal hyperplasia involving 21-hydroxylase deficiency, which of the following is correct?
A. Cortisol accumulates.
B. Levels of ACTH in blood decrease.

C. 17-OH-progesterone is an effective treatment.
D. Pregnenolone synthesis is depressed.
E. Most patients suffer “salt wasting” due to lack of aldosterone.

24. You are seeing a 7-year-old inner-city child with suspected lead poisoning. Because you realize that lead poisoning inhibits ALA dehydrase, you would expect to see an elevated level of
A. succinyl CoA
B. glycine
C. bilirubin
D. ∂-aminolevulinic acid
E. heme

25. All of the following are correct features of nucleotides **except** that they are
A. monomeric units of nucleic acids
B. physiologic mediators
C. sources of chemical energy
D. structural components of membranes
E. structural components of coenzymes

26. Which of the following statements accurately describes features of **cystinosis**?
A. Patients excrete massive amounts of cystine.
B. Mental retardation ensues at an early age.
C. Crystals of cystine are deposited in many tissues.
D. Patient’s growth is retarded.
E. Pancreas and brain are the most affected organs.

27. In chronic myeloid leukemia (CML), the entire abl oncogene is translocated from its normal position on chromosome 9 to chromosome 22. Which of the following treatments has proven to be effective in curing patients with CML?
A. 5-fluorouracil
B. busulfan
C. interferon
D. bone marrow transplantation
E. antisense oligonucleotides

28. Which of the following pairs of codons is **least likely** to code for two different amino acids?
A. UCG : UCA
B. UAC : UAU
C. UAC : AUC
D. UAC : CUA
E. UAC : ACU

29. Cyanide blocks mitochondrial respiration by
A. inhibiting the F_0F_1-ATPase
B. inhibiting the ADP-ATP translocase
C. reacting with heme a on cytochrome oxidase

D. reacting with copper on cytochrome oxidase
E. reacting with heme c on cytochrome c

30. Which of the following serves as a precursor for testosterone?
A. aldosterone
B. cholesterol
C. cortisol
D. estrone
E. none of these

31. During reperfusion of ischemic myocardium, which of the following substrates is required for the burst of free radical production?
A. glutathione
B. ATP
C. molecular oxygen
D. creatine kinase
E. vitamin E

32. The enzyme that catalyzes the reaction

acetoacetate + succinyl CoA ↔ acetoacetyl CoA + succinate

is essentially absent in
A. cardiac muscle
B. striated muscle
C. brain
D. liver
E. kidney

33. Pathways common to many tissues include all of the following **except**
A. glycolysis
B. glycogenolysis
C. lipolysis
D. production of NADPH from glucose 6-phosphate
E. ketogenesis

34. In the normal state of a human at rest, the largest share of blood glucose used as fuel is consumed in the
A. adipose tissue
B. brain
C. kidneys
D. liver
E. muscle

35. The deficient enzyme in von Gierke's disease is
A. hepatic phosphorylase
B. catalase
C. glucose 6-phosphatase
D. glycogen phosphorylase
E. phenylalanine hydroxylase

36. You are working in a medical clinic in a third-world country where most of your patients are in some stage of starvation. Of the following, the substance you would expect to be most depleted in the blood and tissues of your patients is
    A. epinephrine
    B. glucagon
    C. glycogen
    D. ketone bodies
    E. norepinephrine

37. All of the following are potential causes of hypoglycemia **except**
    A. liver disease
    B. excessive alcohol consumption
    C. some adenocarcinomas
    D. glycogen storage diseases
    E. pyruvate kinase deficiency

38. During gluconeogenesis, alanine, and lactate are converted to
    A. acetyl CoA
    B. aspartate
    C. malate
    D. oxaloacetate
    E. pyruvate

39. The diagram below depicts the synthesis of DNA. When strand C starts being synthesized, what other piece is being synthesized?
    A. strand A
    B. strand B
    C. strand D
    D. strand E
    E. No other strand is simultaneously synthesized.

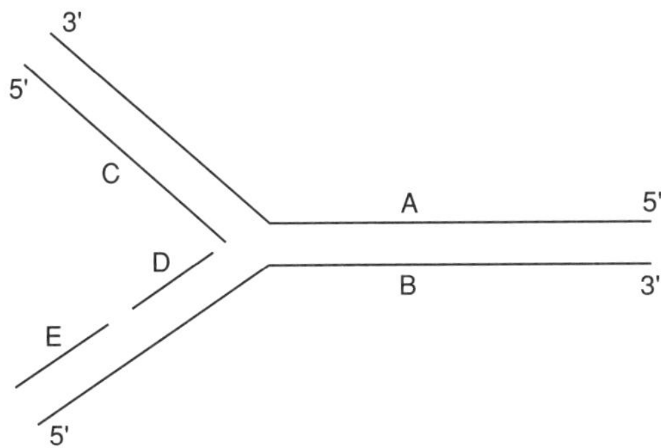

40. The concentration of a particular enzyme was increased to 50 times normal. Which of the following correctly describes the impact this will have on the equilibrium constant of the reaction which that enzyme catalyzes?
    A. It will increase by a factor of 5.
    B. It will decrease by a factor of 5.
    C. It will increase proportionately.

D. It will increase 50-fold.
E. It will be unchanged.

Items 41–43

Match each descriptive statement regarding RNA synthesis inhibitors to the appropriate term. Each lettered choice may be used once, more than once, or not at all.

A. actinomycin D
B. acyclovir
C. rifampin
D. streptomycin
E. tetracycline

41. Binds to bacterial RNA polymerase and prevents initiation of RNA synthesis.
42. Binds to bacterial RNA polymerase; prevents elongation of RNA chains.
43. When it is present, DNA cannot act as a template for transcription.

Items 44–48

Match each of the following descriptions of abnormal states to the substance with which it is most closely associated. Each lettered choice may be used once, more than once, or not at all.

A. folic acid
B. niacin
C. vitamin A
D. vitamin B_1
E. vitamin B_2
F. vitamin B_6
G. vitamin B_{12}
H. vitamin C
I. vitamin D
J. vitamin E
K. vitamin K

44. A collective term for retinol, retinal, and retinoic acid; important in the biochemistry of vision.
45. Probably the most common vitamin deficiency in the US; can produce megaloblastic anemia.
46. Prolonged administration of large doses can produce hemolytic anemia and jaundice in infants.
47. Primary function is as an antioxidant; vegetable oils are a rich source.
48. Whole wheat bread is a good source; a deficiency is seen in association with chronic alcoholism.

Explanations for Biochemistry Items

1. A

2. A

3. C

4. D (Stryer 1988, 830–831). The generation time of the eukaryotic cell can be divided into four stages: mitosis (cell division), G1 (gap 1, before DNA synthesis), S (period of DNA synthesis), and G2 (gap 2, between DNA synthesis and mitosis). The sum of the four phases is equivalent to the generation time. Therefore, the length of DNA synthesis would be 14 hours (i.e., 24 – 6 – 3 – 1 = 14).

5. D (Stryer 1988, 678–679). Xeroderma pigmentosum is an autosomal recessive trait in which the skin of an affected homozygote is extremely sensitive to sunlight. As a consequence of the ultraviolet radiation, pyrimidine dimers are formed in the DNA. The normal repair mechanism, consisting of a DNA endonuclease responsible for hydrolyzing the pyrimidine dimer, has been shown to be defective. As a result, the patient often dies of skin cancer before age 30, unless the skin is carefully shielded from sunlight. Enzyme therapy would be ineffective since the disease has also been shown to be caused by mutations in eight other genes involved in DNA repair.

6. C

7. A (Stryer 1988, 18–21, 28–30). The three predominant forces that determine a protein's three-dimensional structure are electrostatic interactions, hydrogen bonds, and hydrophobic interactions. In a globular protein, the protein is folded such that hydrogen bonding and electrostatic interactions occur on the surface, where the protein is in contact with water, while nonpolar residues are tightly packed in the interior of the molecule, forming necessary hydrophobic interactions that stabilize the tertiary structure. Therefore, aspartic acid, glutamic acid, histidine, and lysine would all be expected to reside on the exterior of the molecule, and alanine, a hydrophobic residue, would be located in the interior of the globular protein.

8. C (Stryer 1988, 154–158). Extensive studies have shown that the deoxyhemoglobin molecule undergoes a change in its conformation upon binding to oxygen. 2,3-Diphosphoglycerate has been shown to bind hemoglobin, having a large effect on its oxygen-binding ability. Hemoglobin consists of an $\alpha_2\beta_2$ structure, with a binding pocket for 2,3-DPG located between the subunits. A person who resides at high altitudes such as the Himalayas would be expected to have elevated levels of 2,3-DPG to compensate for the lower partial pressure of oxygen. Therefore, the oxygen-binding curve is more sigmoidal in the presence of 2,3-DPG, which allows hemoglobin to release oxygen more readily in the tissues.

9. A

10. D

11. E

12. A (Stryer 1988, 508–509). The B vitamins are essential water-soluble

micronutrients. Humans are not capable of synthesizing the B vitamins, and therefore must obtain them from their diet. The absorption of complex B vitamins can be inhibited by various drugs including alcohol. Some vitamins, including vitamin B_{12}, are absorbed by a special transport system that is secreted in the stomach and is subsequently transferred to the intestinal lumen. Furthermore, vitamin B_{12} is unique in that it can only be synthesized by microorganisms. Nutrition deficiencies of vitamin B_{12} are rare since this vitamin can be found in virtually all animal tissues. However, strict vegetarianism can lead to pernicious anemia, which is caused by deficiencies of vitamin B_{12}.

13. D

14. D

15. D

16. A (Stryer 1988, 244–246). The digestive enzyme trypsin is synthesized by the exocrine cells of the pancreas in an enzymatically inactive zymogen known as trypsinogen. The activation of trypsinogen to form trypsin is performed by enterokinase, which is a proteolytic enzyme secreted by the intestinal cells. Enterokinase hydrolyzes a unique lysine-isoleucine peptide bond of trypsinogen as it enters the duodenum from the pancreas. The active trypsin can then go to on to convert additional trypsinogen into trypsin as well as activate additional protease zymogens required for digestion, including proelastase, procarboxypeptidase, and chymotrypsinogen. Thus, the activation of trypsinogen into trypsin is the first step required for digestion. Trypsin hydrolyzes the peptide bonds whose carbonyl groups are either lysine (K) or arginine (R).

17. E (Stryer 1988, 578–579). Essential amino acids are those that cannot be synthesized and thus need to be supplied by the diet. Nine of the twenty natural amino acids are essential for humans, including histidine, isoleucine, leucine, lysine, methionine, phenylalanine, threonine, tryptophan, and valine. The remaining nonessential amino acids can be synthesized by the body from many metabolic precursors, including essential amino acids. For example, phenylalanine, an essential amino acid, undergoes a parahydroxylation to form tyrosine, a nonessential amino acid. Essential amino acids can also be used for synthesis of neurotransmitters. Tyrosine undergoes multiple oxidative steps to form epinephrine, while tryptophan is a precursor for serotonin.

18. B

19. E (Stryer 1988, 502). In the urea cycle, Co_2, NH_4^+, and aspartate are converted to urea and fumarate, at the expense of three ATP molecules. Fumarate is an important intermediate of the citric acid cycle, and can therefore be converted to oxaloacetate. A further transamination reaction of oxaloacetate can convert oxaloacetate to aspartate, providing an additional link between the two cycles.

20. E (Stryer 1988, 30, 40). The three predominant forces that determine a protein's three-dimensional structure are electrostatic interactions, hydrogen bonds, and hydrophobic interactions. While all three are important for a protein's tertiary structure, hydrophobic interactions play the largest role in protein folding. Since proteins exist in a predominantly aqueous environment, the strong tendency for hydrophobic residues to associate together to flee from water drives the folding of a soluble protein. Nonpolar residues are tightly packed in the interior of the molecule, forming necessary hydrophobic interactions that stabilize the tertiary structure.

21. D (Stryer 1988, 150–156). Hemoglobin is a tetrameric $\alpha_{2\beta}2$ protein while myoglobin is a monomeric (α) protein. Structural analysis has revealed that, while there is very little primary sequence similarity between the two proteins, the tertiary structures display striking similarities. Hemoglobin and myoglobin each contain one heme molecule per subunit, consisting of an iron atom that is identical in both coordination and oxidation states. The binding of oxygen to hemoglobin has been shown to be sigmoidal, indicating that the binding of the first oxygen molecule facilitates the binding of the second oxygen molecule, and the cycle continues until all four oxygen molecules are bound. Myoglobin, on the other hand, has a hyperbolic-shaped oxygen-binding curve, consistent with the fact that myoglobin is monomeric and cannot bind oxygen cooperatively.

22. A

23. B

24. D

25. D (Stryer 1988, 316–320, 455, 458, 617–618, 976–978). Nucleotides, which are monomeric units of nucleic acids, play key roles in almost all biochemical pathways. They are activated precursors of both DNA and RNA molecules. Nucleotides are phosphorylated at one of the pentose hydroxyl groups, and therefore can be hydrolyzed for the production of energy. Both ATP, the universal energy carrier, and GTP can act as sources of power for a variety of biochemical mechanisms. Coenzymes such as NAD^+ and CoA contain the nucleotide adenine as part of their complex structure. Cyclic AMP, derived from ATP, is a ubiquitous physiological mediator for numerous cellular reactions.

26. C

27. D

28. D

29. C (Stryer 1988, 412–413). Electron flow in mitochondrial respiration can be blocked by a variety of inhibitors. Cytochrome oxidase mediates the transfer of electrons from cytochrome c to O_2. Four electrons must

flow to O_2 in order for H_2O to be formed in a very complex reaction carried out by cytochrome oxidase. Three inhibitors, CN^-, N_3^- and CO, all stop the electron flow by reacting with cytochrome oxidase. Cytochrome oxidase consists of two molecules of tightly bound heme α along with two essential copper atoms. All three inhibitors bind to the heme α_3 center found in cytochrome oxidase to stop electron flow to oxygen.

30. B (Stryer 1988, 565–568). Progestagens, glucocorticoids, mineralocorticoids, androgens, and estrogens are the five major classes of steroid hormones. Cholesterol is the precursor for all five classes of these hormones. Testosterone, which is within the androgen class, is an important male sex hormone.

31. C

32. D

33. E

34. B (Stryer 1988, 634–637). The brain requires a continuous supply of glucose for normal operation. Since the brain has no stores of built-up energy, it relies heavily on glucose delivered to it through the blood. The brain consumes approximately 60% of the blood glucose when the body is in a resting state. Muscle cells differ from the brain in that the muscles have a large store of glycogen that can be used to supply energy. In resting muscle, fatty acids are the primary source of fuel. The liver and kidney can utilize keto acids derived from amino acid degradation. In a resting cell, adipose tissue converts glycogen to glucose, making energy available for other cells.

35. C (Stryer 1988, 465). von Gierke's disease is a liver disease in which the patient is unable to break down glycogen. A patient with this disease has an enlarged liver, due to the buildup of glycogen in the liver cells. Furthermore, patients show prolonged hypoglycemia between meals, indicative of an inability to produce glucose from glucose 6-phosphate. Glucose 6-phosphate builds up in the liver since it cannot transverse the membrane, causing an increase in the level of glycolysis. As a consequence, patients have a high level of lactate and pyruvate in the blood. Since lactate is formed from the glycogen but glucose is not, the enzyme that is defective is glucose 6-phosphatase, which converts glucose 6-phosphate to glucose.

36. C

37. E

38. E (Stryer 1988, 444, 504). Lactate is a dead-end molecule formed during glycolysis from the reduction of pyruvate by NADH under anaerobic conditions. Transamination of alanine also leads to lactate. An important step before gluconeogenesis, which is the biosynthesis of new glucose from noncarbohydrate precursors, involves the reoxidation of lactate to form pyruvate. Pyruvate then becomes carboxylated to form oxaloacetate, the first step in gluconeogenesis.

39. C (Stryer 1988, 673). DNA replication occurs at a location commonly referred to as the replication fork (see figure). In this diagram, strand C, the leading strand, is being synthesized in the direction of the fork (to the right), while the most recent lagging strand, strand D, is being synthesized away from the fork (to the left). Strand E is a lagging strand that is no longer being synthesized, and will eventually be connected to strand D by the enzyme DNA ligase.

40. E (Stryer 1988, 183). An enzyme is a biologic catalyst that increases the rate of a reaction by lowering the activation energy required for a reaction to proceed. An equilibrium constant is a thermodynamic property of a reaction relating the specific concentrations of all reactants and products at equilibrium at a given temperature and pressure. The equilibrium constant of a reaction is not dependent upon the reaction rate, and thus will not change by increasing or decreasing the rate of the reaction.

41. C, 42. D, 43. A (Stryer 1988, 714–715). RNA polymerase catalyzes the elongation of RNA molecules from a DNA template strand. Many antibiotics have been shown to inhibit this reaction, thus preventing protein synthesis, which in turn leads to cell termination. Rifampin inhibits the initiation of RNA synthesis by RNA polymerase, and has been used by molecular biologists to determine which transcripts are being newly synthesized without endangering the cell. Another antibiotic, actinomycin D, has been found to intercalate its phenoxazone ring between neighboring base pairs on the DNA template, which inhibits transcription of DNA by RNA polymerase. Therefore, DNA cannot act as a template for RNA polymerase in the presence of actinomycin D. Streptomycin is an aminoglycoside that interferes with the attachment of messenger RNA to ribosomes in the initiation of protein synthesis.

44. C

45. A

46. K

47. J

48. D

Reference

Stryer L: Biochemistry. 3rd ed. New York: Freeman, 1988.

Physiology

1. The movement of a particular ion was found to be directly proportional to the concentration gradient at all concentrations of that ion. From this, one can conclude that the transport process is
   A. active transport

B. facilitated diffusion
C. Na^+ coupled cotransport
D. not possible to determine from these data
E. simple diffusion

Items 2–5

For each statement below, choose the term with which it is most closely associated.

A. preload
B. summation
C. isometric contraction
D. isotonic contraction
E. excitation-contraction (EC) coupling

2. The process by which an action potential initiates a contraction.
3. Muscle contracts against an afterload and shortens.
4. Muscle length remains constant during the contractile event.
5. The increase in muscle force due to repeated stimulation.

6. In the context of the human body, the resting potential of a nerve membrane will depend on the concentration gradient of which of the following ions?
A. bicarbonate
B. calcium
C. chloride
D. potassium
E. sodium

7. In vision, the ability of the eye to accommodate involves all of the following events **except**
A. parasympathetic nerves release acetylcholine
B. ciliary muscle contracts
C. lens ligaments contract
D. lens shape becomes more biconvex
E. All of these statements are correct.

8. Which of the following will determine whether neurotransmitter release at a synaptic junction will excite or inhibit postsynaptic neurons?
A. reuptake rate of neurotransmitter for presynaptic cells
B. the presynaptic axon's speed of axoplasmic transport
C. the chemical composition of the neurotransmitter
D. the postsynaptic cell's properties
E. the absolute amount of calcium released by the presynaptic cells

9. You are treating a patient with medications to increase the contractility of her heart muscle. The decreased contractility of this patient's cardiac muscle could be due to any of the following factors **except**
A. hypoxia
B. acidosis
C. myocardial ischemia

D. infarcts
E. hemorrhage

Items 10–12

The diagram below shows a typical electrocardiogram tracing. Select the numbered segment that fits each description.

10. The segment that reflects atrial depolarization.
11. The segment that reflects ventricular repolarization.
12. Prolongation of this segment can indicate blockage in one of the bundle branches.

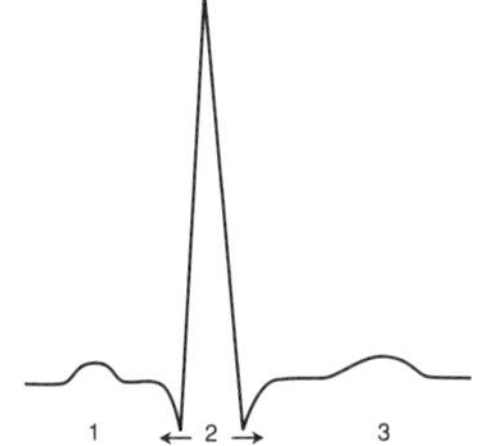

13. A 56-year-old businessman undergoes coronary arteriography, which reveals a 50% decrease in the lumen of one coronary artery. As compared to a nonoccluded artery, flow through this occluded vessel will decrease by a factor of
    A. 4
    B. 8
    C. 12
    D. 16
    E. 24

Items 14–16

The graph shows forced vital capacity maneuvers from three individuals. The Y axis represents the absolute lung volume. TLC = total lung capacity; RV = residual volume. Select the lettered curve that fits each description.

14. This individual appears to have normal lung function.
15. This individual may have emphysema.
16. This individual may have sarcoid.

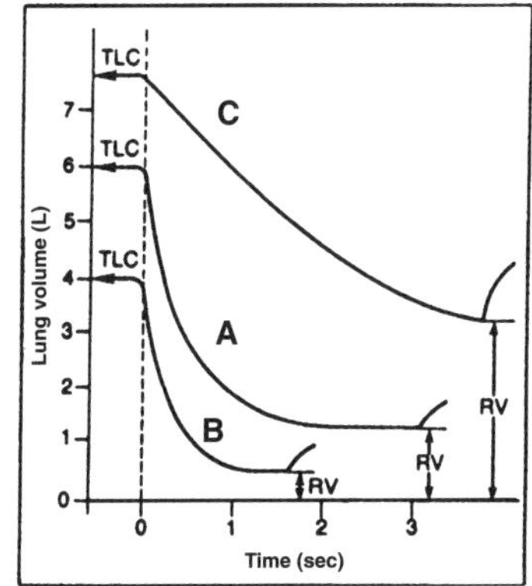

17. In a normal standing person, which of the following contributes to the observation that the ventilation-perfusion ratio is higher at the top of the lungs than at the bottom?
    A. At FRC, transpulmonary pressure is greater at the top than at the bottom.
    B. The lungs are more compliant at the top than at the bottom.
    C. Breathing frequency is higher at the bottom than at the top.
    D. Blood flow is higher at the top than at the bottom.
    E. Regional perfusion is distributed more evenly vertically than is regional ventilation.

Items 18–22

From the diagram below, select the lettered pattern of endocrine changes that best represents each diagnosis. The arrows represent **above** or **below** normal levels.

18. Cushing's disease
19. ectopic ACTH syndrome
20. primary adrenocortical insufficiency
21. secondary adrenocortical insufficiency
22. cortisol-secreting adrenocortical tumor

	Pituitary ACTH secretion	Plasma ACTH	Adrenal cortisol secretion
A	↑	↑	↓
B	↓	↓	↑
C	↓	↓	↓
D	↑	↑	↑
E	↓	↑	↑

23. The extrinsic pathway of the clotting system in humans is activated by a tissue substance composed primarily of
    A. collagen
    B. elastin
    C. glycoprotein
    D. lipoprotein
    E. triglyceride

24. A patient whose serum potassium was elevated to 6 mEq/L also had an abnormal finding on ECG. Which finding is most likely associated with his elevated potassium level?
    A. a decrease in the PR interval
    B. a decrease in the QT interval
    C. high peaked T waves
    D. low-amplitude P waves
    E. shortened QRS duration

25. In a normal person, the fraction of the filtered load of glucose reabsorbed in the proximal convoluted tubule is approximately
    A. 40%
    B. 100%
    C. 25%
    D. 60%
    E. zero

Items 26–28

Refer to the following diagram of a nephron to answer the next three items. Each lettered site may be used once, more than once, or not at all.

26. The largest fraction of filtered load of sodium is reabsorbed at this site.
27. Changes in glomerular filtration rate by alterations in the concentration of sodium chloride are mediated at this site.
28. Significant urea permeability modulated by ADH could be found at this site.

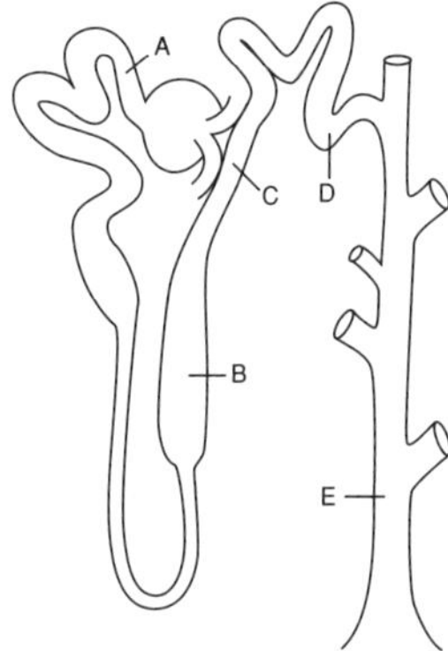

Items 29–31

Match each description to the term with which it is most closely associated. Choices may be used once, more than once, or not at all.

A. glucagon
B. glucose
C. insulin
D. leucine and arginine
E. somatostatin

29. Peptide that directly promotes hepatic glycogen storage.
30. Peptide that directly increases gluconeogenesis.
31. Peptide that inhibits pancreatic alpha- and beta-cell function.

32. Patients with congestive heart failure nearly always suffer from edema. Which of the following factors is most closely linked to the development of edema in these patients?
    A. increased cell membrane K^+ permeability
    B. increased plasma oncotic pressure

C. decreased plasma renin activity
D. sodium retention
E. stimulation of ADH release

33. An increase in blood pressure from 100 to 130 mmHg produces all of the following effects **except**
    A. an increased nerve traffic from arterial baroreceptors
    B. an increase in vagal tone
    C. a decrease in sympathetic tone
    D. an increased diameter of the carotid sinus
    E. a stimulation of vasopressin release

34. A 55-year-old factory worker, complaining of dyspnea, had pulmonary function testing performed at a hospital. The following values were obtained: FVC = 2.45 L, FEV_1 = 1.30 L, TLC = 5.80 L, RV = 2.35 L, FRC = 3.90 L. These results are most consistent with a diagnosis of
    A. chronic emphysema
    B. interstitial pulmonary fibrosis
    C. pleural effusion
    D. pulmonary edema
    E. sarcoidosis

Items 35–38

Match the stage of the menstrual cycle to the lettered event with which it is most closely associated. Choices may be used once, more than once, or not at all.

A. Dominant follicle becomes autonomous.
B. LH surge begins.
C. Corpus luteum "dies."
D. ovulation
E. Menses ends.

35. day 15 of the menstrual cycle
36. day 11 of the menstrual cycle
37. day 7 of the menstrual cycle
38. day 23 of the menstrual cycle

39. A convict has been on a hunger strike for 7 days to protest conditions inside the prison. Which of the following conclusions about his current metabolic state would be justified?
    A. He would show an increased insulin-to-glucagon ratio.
    B. He would show decreased gluconeogenesis.
    C. He would show increased glycogenesis.
    D. He would show increased amino acid uptake in muscle.
    E. He would show none of these effects.

40. A cardiologist informs you that one of your patients has the following findings: The pressure-volume loop of the left ventricle is displaced upward and to the right and exhibits an increase in the loop area. You quickly realize that your patient suffers from

A. aortic stenosis
B. intraventricular septal defect with left-to-right shunt
C. mitral regurgitation
D. mitral stenosis
E. pulmonic stenosis

41. Upon leaving your office late one evening, you realize that you are being followed as you walk toward your car in a deserted parking structure. Because of this threatening situation, sympathetic discharge would be expected to
A. reduce your heart rate
B. reduce your arterial blood pressure
C. increase your cardiac output
D. increase your vagal tone
E. increase your glomerular filtration rate

42. A newborn underwent a procedure to open a blocked lacrimal gland. The lacrimal gland
A. actively reabsorbs K^+, leading to $[K^+] <1$ mEq/L in tears
B. is inhibited by cholinergic stimulation
C. is the primary source of the lipid bilayer in the tear film
D. secretes proteins that have an antibacterial function in tears
E. All of the above statements are correct.

43. The major site of production for cerebrospinal fluid is the
A. arachnoid granulation
B. brain parenchymal capillary endothelial cell
C. choroid plexus capillary endothelial cell
D. choroid plexus epithelial cell
E. glial cell

44. You have been asked to examine the ECG of a patient who was told that he has a complete left bundle branch block. If this diagnosis is correct, which of the following would you expect to see on his ECG?
A. increased amplitude of the T wave
B. inversion of the T wave
C. prolonged duration of QRS
D. prolonged PR interval
E. prolonged QT interval

45. Which of the following most strongly suggests a diagnosis of primary aldosteronism?
A. increased circulating catecholamines
B. increased circulating renin
C. low plasma potassium
D. marked elevation in plasma creatinine concentration
E. pressure gradient between the upper and lower part of the body

46. Hyperprolactinemia leads to amenorrhea primarily by inducing
A. a direct effect of prolactin on the Leydig cell
B. a direct effect of prolactin on the proliferation of the endometrium

C. compression of the pars nervosa
D. hypergonadotrophic hypogonadism
E. hypogonadotrophic hypogonadism

47. You have been treating a 73-year-old patient with moderate emphysema. In this patient
    A. lung compliance is less than normal
    B. the maximum expired flow rate is greater than normal
    C. the residual volume is less than normal
    D. increased breathing frequency makes ventilation distribution more even
    E. obstruction of the airway occurs during expiration

Items 48–50

Match the gastrointestial event to the most appropriate functional description. Each choice may be used once, more than once, or not at all.

A. giant migrating contractions
B. individual phasic contractions
C. migrating motor complexes
D. retrograde giant contractions
E. None of these is correct.

48. Mixes food with secretions and propels the chyme slowly in a caudal direction.
49. Rapidly propels contents of the proximal small intestine into the antrum.
50. Cleans the small intestine of debris and residual food in the interdigestive state.

Explanations for Physiology Items

1. E

2. E

3. D

4. C

5. B

6. D (Kandel et al. 1991, 82–89). The resting nerve cell membrane is permeable to only three ion species: K^+, Na^+, and Cl^-. Chloride ions are in equilibrium due to lack of any Cl^- pump in nerve cells. Thus, Cl^- distributes passively across the cell membrane and does not contribute to resting membrane potential (RPM). K^+ and Na^+ are not in equilibrium in a resting nerve cell, but rather in a steady state due to the action of the

Na^+-K^+ pump. The resting nerve cell membrane is 100 times more permeable to K^+ than to Na^+. Thus, RPM is determined mainly by the concentration gradient for K^+, approximates the equilibrium potential for K^+, and can be predicted at different K^+ gradients by the Nernst equation. At low K^+ gradients, the membrane potential deviates from the value predicted by the Nernst potential for K^+, indicating the involvement of Na^+, which, despite the low permeability, still has a finite net flux because of the large Na^+ gradient across the cell membrane.

7. C (Ganong 1993, 137). The process by which the curvature of the lens is increased is called accommodation. At rest, the lens is held under tension by the lens ligaments. Because the lens substance is malleable and the lens capsule has considerable elasticity, the lens is pulled into a flattened shape. When the gaze is directed at a near object, the ciliary muscle contracts. This decreases the distance between the edges of the ciliary body and relaxes the lens ligaments, so that the lens springs into a more convex shape.

8. D (Kandel et al. 1991, 132). The action of a specific chemical messenger in the postsynaptic cell does not depend on the chemical nature of the transmitter, but instead on the properties of the receptors with which the transmitter binds. For example, acetylcholine can excite some postsynaptic cells and inhibit others, and can do both simultaneously at still others. It is the receptor that determines whether a cholinergic synapse is excitatory or inhibitory.

9. E

10. 1

11. 3

12. 2

13. D (Guyton 1991, 156). According to Poiseuille's law, the rate of blood flow is directly proportional to the fourth power of the radius of the vessel. A 2-fold change in vessel diameter changes blood flow 16-fold.

14. B

15. C

16. A

17. A

18. D, 19. E, 20. A, 21. C, 22. B (Ganong 1993, 342–347). Depending on plasma cortisol levels, the clinical syndromes of adrenocortical dysfunction can be classified into hypo- and hypersecretion of cortisol. Cortisol hyposecretion syndromes include primary and secondary adrenocortical insufficiencies. In primary insufficiency, the primary defect is in the

adrenal gland itself, which leads to increased pituitary secretion of ACTH due to the release of feedback inhibition. In secondary insufficiency, the defect is in the pituitary, leading to low levels of ACTH and secondary hyposecretion of cortisol. All other syndromes are examples of adrenocortical hyperfunction where cortisol levels are high. Cushing's disease is a primary pituitary ACTH hypersecretion; thus, the plasma levels of both ACTH and cortisol are high. Plasma levels of both ACTH and cortisol are also high in ectopic ACTH syndrome, where ACTH is being produced by a tissue other than the pituitary and exerts a negative feedback on pituitary ACTH release. Finally, cortisol-secreting adrenocortical tumor is characterized by high cortisol, which exhibits a negative feedback inhibition on pituitary ACTH release, leading to low plasma levels.

23. D (Ganong 1993, 490). The extrinsic pathway for clotting is triggered by the release of tissue thromboplastin (factor III), a protein-phospholipid mixture that activates factor VII. Tissue thromboplastin and factor VII activate factors IX and X. In the presence of platelet phospholipid, Ca^{2+}, and factor V, activated factor X catalyzes the conversion of prothrombin to thrombin.

24. C (Ganong 1993, 509). Hyperkalemia, plasma potassium ion concentration higher than 5.5 mEq/L, is a very dangerous and potentially lethal condition because of its effects on the heart. As plasma K^+ level rises, the first change in the ECG is the appearance of tall peaked T waves, a manifestation of altered repolarization.

25. B (Ganong 1993, 646). Normally, glucose is filtered at a rate of approximately 100 mg per minute (80 mg/dl normal plasma glucose $\times$ 125 ml/min normal GFR). Glucose is reabsorbed by secondary active transport along with Na^+ in the early portion of the proximal tubule. The amount reabsorbed is proportionate to the amount filtered up to the transport maximum (Tm) for glucose, which is 375 mg per minute for men and 300 mg per minute for women. Thus, in a normal person, 100% of the filtered load of glucose is reabsorbed back.

26. A (Berne and Levy 1993, 743). Proximal tubule reabsorption of Na^+ occurs across the paracellular pathway and across the trascellular pathway. Approximately 17,000 mEq of the 25,000 mEq of sodium filtered each day is reabsorbed in the proximal tubule (67% of the filtered load).

27. B (Berne and Levy 1993, 737). Autoregulation of renal blood flow and GFR is thought to be a function of two mechanisms: the myogenic mechanism and the tubuloglomerular feedback. The latter involves a feedback loop in which the flow of tubular fluid (or some other factor, such as the rate of NaCl reabsorption, which increases in direct proportion to flow) is sensed by the macula densa in the thick ascending limb of Henle's loop and is converted into a signal that affects GFR.

28. E (Berne and Levy 1993, 765). In the presence of ADH, the reabsorption of water from the tubular fluid across the cortical and outer medullary

portions of the collecting duct causes the urea concentration to rise. When this fluid reaches the inner medullary collecting duct, urea diffuses out of the tubule into the interstitium.

29. C

30. A

31. E

32. D (Guyton 1991, 249). After the first day or so of cardiac failure, peripheral edema begins to develop because of fluid retention by the kidneys. The retention of fluid increases the mean systemic filling pressure, resulting in increased tendency for blood to return to the heart with subsequent increase in cardiac output and arterial pressure. There are three know causes of the reduced renal output of urine during cardiac failure: (1) decreased glomerular filtration, (2) activation of the renin-angiotensin system and increased reabsorption of water and salt by the renal tubules, and (3) increased aldosterone secretion.

33. E (Guyton 1991, 198, 829). An increase in arterial blood pressure leads to an increased frequency of transmission of impulses from arterial baroreceptors. The signal enters the tractus solitarius of the medulla and leads to the generation of secondary signals that inhibit the vasoconstrictor center of the medulla and excite the vagal center. The net effects are vasodilation throughout the peripheral circulatory system, including the carotid sinus itself, and decreased heart rate and contractility with subsequent rapid decrease of arterial pressure. Vasopressin release is inhibited by increased stretch of the baroreceptors.

34. A (Guyton 1991, 455–456). The FEV_1/FVC ratio is less than the normal value of 80%, which suggests a chronic obstructive pulmonary disease (COPD). All other options, except chronic emphysema, are examples of a chronic restrictive pulmonary disease (CRPD). This is also suggested by the higher than normal values of RV and FRC, which is characteristic of COPD, but inconsistent with what would be expected in CRPD.

35. D

36. B

37. A

38. C

39. E

40. A

41. C

42. D

43. D

44. C

45. C

46. E

47. E

48. B

49. D

50. C

References

Berne RM, Levy MN: Physiology, 3rd ed. St. Louis: Mosby, 1993.

Ganong WF: Review of Medical Physiology. 16th ed. Norwalk, CT: Appleton & Lange, 1993.

Guyton AC: Textbook of Medical Physiology. 8th ed. Philadelphia: Saunders, 1991.

Kandel ER, Schwartz JH, Jessel TM: Principles of Neural Science. 3rd ed. New York: Elsevier, 1991.

Behavioral Sciences

1. You are seeing a 63-year-old woman for the first time. She is brought in by her daughter, who is concerned about her mother's memory lapses and displays of poor judgment for the past year. In addition to these problems, she reports that her mother has become incontinent and has been walking oddly for the past 3 months. Which of the following should definitely be on your list of differential diagnoses?
   A. depression
   B. Parkinson's disease
   C. cerebrovascular vasoconstriction
   D. normal-pressure hydrocephalus
   E. malnutrition

2. Which of the following statements regarding alcohol (ETOH) abuse in the elderly is **incorrect**?
   A. Elderly alcoholics often present with complaints not typical of ETOH abuse.

B. Depression is a common corollary to ETOH abuse in the elderly.
C. Incontinence is suggestive of ETOH abuse in the elderly.
D. Older alcoholics tend to be more hostile than younger alcoholics.
E. Diarrhea and frequent falls may indicate that an ETOH problem is present.

Items 3–7

Match each definition statement to the term with which it is most closely associated. The lettered choices may be used once, more than once, or not at all.

A. bias
B. interval scale
C. median
D. mean
E. measurement error
F. mode
G. nominal scale
H. ordinal scale
I. range
J. relative frequency
K. variance
L. standard deviation

3. This index is calculated by taking the average of the squared deviations around the mean.
4. The middle value of a sample of observations arranged by magnitude.
5. This is defined as the number of observations falling into each interval of an interval scale.
6. This is comprised of a limited number of categories that cannot be arranged in a hierarchical manner.
7. This is the systematic component of variation, both in nature and in measurement.

8. Values of a certain enzyme were determined by hospital laboratory personnel during routine hospitalizations of 1000 patients. The distribution of these data was normal, with an enzyme level mean of 18.5 units and a standard deviation of 3.5 units. Which of the following is a valid conclusion from these data?
   A. The most frequently measured level of the enzyme was 18.5 units.
   B. About half of the patients had enzyme levels in the range of 18.0 to 19.0 units.
   C. An enzyme level of greater than 22.0 would be abnormal.
   D. Ninety-five percent of the enzyme values fell between 8.0 and 25.5 units.
   E. Fifty percent of the enzyme values fell between 15.0 and 22.0 units.

Items 9–12

Match each of the statements below to the appropriate psychoactive substance. Each lettered choice may be used once, more than once, or not at all.

A. amphetamines
B. caffeine
C. cannabis
D. cocaine
E. inhalants
F. nicotine
G. opioids
H. sedatives/hypnotics/anxiolytics

9. Both methadone and clonidine have been used successfully in treatment.
10. Most lethal psychoactive substance that is not illegal.
11. Complications include hepatotoxicity, neurotoxicity, cardiac arrhythmias, and methemoglobulinemia.
12. May cause a paranoid psychosis similar to schizophrenia.

13. Which of the following statements about schizophrenia is **incorrect**?
    A. The incidence is about 1–2% in the general population.
    B. Siblings of schizophrenics are not significantly more at risk of developing schizophrenia than unrelated persons.
    C. The disorder is believed to result, at least partly, from a hyperdopaminergic state.
    D. Haloperidol can be an effective treatment.

Items 14–15

Match each of the following statements about disorders with a genetic component to the appropriate term. Each lettered choice may be used once, more than once, or not at all.

A. alcohol abuse
B. Alzheimer's disease
C. attention deficit disorder
D. bipolar disorder
E. Hartnup disease
F. Huntington's chorea
G. schizophrenia
H. Tourette's syndrome
I. unipolar disorder

14. Simple and complex motor tics, sometimes with coprolalia, which usually begin in childhood.
15. Due to dysfunction in the transport of neutral amino acids, characterized by emotional lability, psychotic episodes, and mental retardation.

16. Which of the following statements **would not** explain a large margin of error in cognitive ability test scores?
    A. reliability coefficient of .60
    B. variance in the testing conditions from one subject to another
    C. differences in interpreting test directions among examinees
    D. inadequate norm group size
    E. natural variation in the population to be tested

17. A 31-year-old woman is seeing you for the first time. She states that in the past 2 months, she has experienced 10 episodes of a bizarre group of symptoms that came without reason, lasted about 30 to 45 minutes, and then gradually diminished. She states that the symptoms included difficulty in breathing, sweating, palpitations, trembling all over, and a feeling that she was choking. She denies any prior psychiatric problems or drug use and says that she passed a thorough physical exam 2 weeks ago "with flying colors." Among the following, which diagnostic possibility is most consistent with her symptoms?
    A. borderline personality disorder
    B. conversion disorder

C. depression
D. panic disorder
E. schizophrenia

18. A young patient is brought in by her mother, who states that the child was bitten by a neighborhood dog several months ago and that the 4-year-girl is now refusing to go to friends' houses if they have cats or dogs and recently became hysterical during a family outing to a petting zoo. The child's behavior is an instance of
A. adaptation
B. confrontation
C. denial
D. stimulus generalization
E. undoing

Items 19–20

For each behavioral description, select the most appropriate age range according to Piaget's theory of cognitive development. Each lettered choice may be used once, more than once, or not at all.

A. birth to 1 month
B. 9 months to 1 year
C. 4–7 years
D. 7–11 years
E. adolescence to maturity

19. There is an increasing capacity for symbolic thought and an ability to classify by similarities and differences.
20. Characterized by formal operations; logical planning and purely abstract thought are now possible.

21. Mortality is rising most rapidly for which of the following age ranges?
A. birth to 4 years
B. 5–11 years
C. 12–20 years
D. 25–40 years
E. 55–75 years

22. A television commercial depicting an attractive, well-dressed woman receiving a diamond bracelet from a handsome, well-dressed man employs which one of the following learning principles?
A. autoshaping
B. classic conditioning
C. imprinting
D. subliminal communication
E. habituation

23. In animals, aggression may be elicited by all of the following **except**
A. stimulation of the hypothalamus of cats
B. lesions of the amygdala

C. pain
D. a threat to offspring
E. the Klüver-Bucy syndrome

24. Etiologic factors in male sexual dysfunction may include all of the following **except**
    A. anxiety
    B. diabetes
    C. phobias
    D. small amounts of alcohol
    E. sympathetic blocking agents

25. Which of the following statements about families is true?
    A. The majority (90%) of the US population lives with relatives.
    B. About one third of those who divorce in the US eventually remarry.
    C. Premarital pregnancy is not a risk factor for divorce.
    D. Single-parent families now comprise more than 40% of all families.
    E. Sixty percent of all murders occur among family members.

26. According to sociologist Talcott Parsons, the "sick role" that society assigns to the ill person consists of all of the following expectations **except**
    A. the sick person is exempt from normal social/role responsibilities
    B. the sick person is not to blame for the illness
    C. the sick person must want to get well
    D. the sick person is allowed to be passive
    E. the sick person must seek competent medical help

Items 27–30

Match each physician statement to the appropriate communication technique. Each lettered choice may be used once, more than once, or not at all.

A. clarification
B. confrontation
C. direct question
D. empathy
E. facilitation
F. interpretation
G. reflection
H. silence
I. summation
J. support

27. "Do you feel the stomach pain you've described for me before or after meals?"
28. "Can you tell me a little more about the type of pain you say you've been experiencing every night?"
29. "I can see that you are really concerned about the surgery you are going to have next week."
30. "You say that you are really afraid of getting lung cancer and yet your wife tells me you are still smoking."

31. Which of the following pairs is an **incorrect** matching of Freud's and Erikson's stages of development?

	Freud	**Erikson**
A.	oral	trust vs. mistrust
B.	anal	autonomy vs. shame, guilt
C.	phallic	industry vs. inferiority
D.	genital	ego identity vs. role diffusion

E. All of these are correctly matched.

32. Which of the following developmental theorists is most likely to have made the following statement?

Each life cycle is characterized by events or crises which must be mastered satisfactorily for optimal development. If mastery of a particular stage is not achieved, all subsequent stages will reflect that deficiency in the form of physical, cognitive, social, or emotional maladjustment.

A. Alfred Adler
B. Erik Erikson
C. Sigmund Freud
D. C. G. Jung
E. B. F. Skinner

33. A young woman is being seen for the first time on a referral from a shelter for battered women. In response to your inquiry about her childhood, she states that her father beat her routinely and she always felt powerless to escape from him. As to her marriage, she insists that her husband was a large, muscular man who could easily dominate her, and therefore she "just took it" until a friend "rescued" her. This woman's response to violence illustrates which of the following behavioral patterns?
A. autoshaping
B. conditioned neurosis
C. displacement behavior
D. learned helplessness
E. splitting

34. A mother has encouraged her young child to cooperate in going to bed by offering to read him a story and then giving him a snack. While this worked well for several months, the mother now seeks your advice as the child has recently resumed tantrum behavior once the story and snack are finished. Which statement best explains this development?
A. The reward reinforced the behavior it followed.
B. Continuous reinforcement eventually led to extinction of the learned behavior.
C. Fear of punishment was extinguished by the reward method.
D. Stimulus generalization resulted in the child identifying the snack with the tantrums.
E. The reward tactic failed because the child is at a preoperational stage of development.

Items 35–38

Match the following examples of impaired forms of speech to the appropriate terms. Each lettered choice may be used once, more than once, or not at all.

A. blocking
B. circumstantiality
C. clang associations
D. confabulation
E. derailment
F. echolalia
G. flight of ideas
H. neologisms
I. perseveration
J. reduced content
K. tangentiality
L. word salad

35. "Yes, I like this place! Do you eat green peppers with a soup spoon?"
36. "The sky is marmaladey and I feel saddlesoaring."
37. "Came why to Johnny and then not. Did when George ate she."
38. "Yes, I'm happy today. . .mayday. . .payday. . .daycare. . .careful. . ."

39. Which of the following is **not** among the "four As" proposed as hallmarks of schizophrenia by Eugene Bleuler?
    A. affect
    B. aggression
    C. ambivalence
    D. association
    E. autism

40. Identify the **incorrect** statement regarding sexual function.
    A. The most common causes of decreased sexual activity following myocardial infarctions are psychological.
    B. Chronic renal failure results in a high incidence of sexual dysfunction.
    C. Only 10% of patients will initiate discussion on sexual function but 50% will discuss the topic if asked by their physician.
    D. Transsexualism is characterized by a belief that the individual belongs to the opposite sex.
    E. The most common cause of vaginismus is medications that block sympathetic nervous system function.

Items 41–44

Match the following descriptions of health care arrangements to the most appropriate term. Each lettered choice may be used once, more than once, or not at all.

A. nonprofit, private insurance carrier
B. for-profit, commercial insurer
C. public insurer
D. health maintenance organization
E. preferred provider organization

41. Physicians contracting to provide service to a specific group of patients.
42. Blue Cross/Blue Shield often serves as a fiscal intermediary for government programs.

43. Subscribers pay an annual premium in exchange for a prearranged package of benefits.
44. Medicaid is a federal- and state-sponsored program that pays the health care expenses of the indigent.

45. Which of the following **is not** an accurate statement regarding patients' responses to being told they have a terminal illness?
    A. Pain control without significant side effects is possible in 30% of patients.
    B. Denial and self-preoccupation are typical early reactions.
    C. Almost all decide against suicide if social support and pain control are provided.
    D. More than half will develop adjustment disorders.
    E. Previous life adjustment is a major factor in determining patients' responses.

46. In response to stress, all of the following physiologic variables show increased levels **except**
    A. antibody production
    B. blood pressure
    C. cortisol
    D. blood fatty acids
    E. blood glucose

Items 47–49

Match the following descriptions of human behavior to the appropriate term. Each lettered choice may be used once, more than once, or not at all.

A. compulsion
B. delusion
C. depersonalization
D. hallucination
E. illusion

47. A wealthy middle-aged woman is discovered to have stolen thousands of articles from local stores. Over 500 jars of cold cream and nearly 800 bottles of nail polish remover were recovered from her home. When asked by detectives why she needed so many, she replied, "I just had to have them."
48. During detoxification, a 49-year-old chronic alcoholic began tearing at his clothing and cringing at the edge of his bed, shouting that millions of spiders were trying to eat him alive.
49. Despite repeated attempts to convince her that she is mistaken, a young woman insists that she is the wife of President Clinton and demands to be taken into the White House immediately by the security staff who are restraining her. She has been arrested on three previous occasions for attempting to enter the White House through the press entrance.

50. All of the following statements accurately characterize patients who suffer from anorexia nervosa **except**

A. white females of upper socioeconomic class have the highest incidence
B. up to 10% will eventually die from the disease or complications stemming from it
C. the disease is thought to involve genetic factors that determine the size and number of fat cells in the body
D. patients with the disease were often "model children" and perfectionists as adults
E. virtually 100% suffer amenorrhea

Explanations for Behavioral Sciences Items

1. D (Simons and Pardes 1981, 459). Normal-pressure hydrocephalus presents with the triad of urinary incontinence, mild dementia, and a typical CT scan showing enlargement of the lateral ventricles with little cortical atrophy. Shunting is frequently successful in eliminating the incontinence and dementia. The dementia and abnormal gait suggest an organic impairment that should be ruled out before psychiatric diagnoses are considered.

2. D

3. K, 4. C, 5. J, 6. G, 7. A (Dawson-Saunders and Trapp 1990, 6–63). Variance is the average of the summed deviations around the mean, calculated by the formula $\Sigma(x–x)/n–1$. Taking the square root of this quantity gives the standard deviation. A nominal scale is used to sample data where the possibilities are limited and nonnumerical, such as when a risk factor is either "present" or "absent." Bias is described as systematic because it influences results in a nonrandom fashion.

8. D

9. G

10. F

11. E

12. D

13. B (Kaplan and Sadock 1988, 108–109). The closer the genetic relationship of any person to a family member affected with schizophrenia, the more likely that person is to develop the disease; for example, among dizygotic twins of schizophrenics, the incidence is 12% as compared to an incidence of 1 to 2% in the general population.

14. H

15. E

16. E

17. D (Simons and Pardes 1981, 169). The diagnostic criteria for panic disorder require at least four attacks within a 4-week period and the sudden development of at least 4 of a list of 13 possible symptoms, including dyspnea, sweating, trembling, choking, and palpitations.

18. D (Simons and Pardes 1981, 553). Stimulus generalization occurs when a stimulus reasonably similar to the original stimulus also produces the learned response. The fear experienced by the child as a result of the dog bite has become generalized to include other four-legged mammals with fur.

19. C, 20. E (Wiener 1987, 96–97). Piaget characterized ages 4 to 7 as the stage of intuitive thought, where children have an increased capacity for symbolic thought and the ability to classify how things are alike and different. It is intuitive because the child may not be able to explain how he or she correctly classified an object. Increasingly after age 12, consequences can be anticipated and therefore logic and advance planning can occur. This is the stage in which purely abstract thought becomes possible.

21. C

22. B (Wiener 1987, 80–84). Imprinting occurs only in birds, shortly after hatching. Autoshaping occurs for responses closely linked to the reinforcement (e.g., food). For example, pecking behavior is reinforced by food in pigeons. Subliminal images can affect responses but the question provided no information on the use of such images in this commercial. Habituation refers to the gradual diminishment of a learned response. After many associations between physical attractiveness/wealth and the product (jewelry in this case), it is hoped that the viewer will correlate buying jewelry with being well-off and attractive, and therefore be more prone to purchase the item. This is classic conditioning, as Pavlov's bell ultimately elicited salivation from the dog without food being present.

23. E (Kaplan and Sadock 1988, 453). Aggression has been experimentally elicited by stimulating the hypothalamus of cats and has also been correlated with lesions of the amygdala. Pain and threats of offspring also trigger aggressive behavior. The Klüver-Bucy syndrome is characterized by the inability to ignore any stimulus, visual agnosia, placidity, hypersexuality, and altered dietary habits, particularly hyperphagia.

24. D

25. A (Wiener 1987, 176). Ninety percent of the US population lives with relatives. Eighty percent of those who divorce remarry. About 20% of US families are single-parent families, and 25% of all murders occur among family members. Premarital pregnancy is one of a number of studied risk factors for divorce. Other risk factors include a short court-

ship, marriage at an early age, and continuing parental opposition to the marriage.

26. D

27. C

28. E

29. D

30. B

31. C

32. B

33. D (Kaplan and Sadock 1988, 141; Wiener 1987, 81–90). Animals who were repeatedly exposed to electric shocks from which they could not escape eventually gave up and made no attempt to avoid future shocks. In humans who are depressed, one finds a similar pattern of learned helplessness. Autoshaping refers to responses closely associated with reinforcements. A conditioned neurosis can be created when a discrimination task is made too difficult. Displacement occurs when animals are prevented from performing a primary behavior such as reproductive behavior. When prohibited, the animal may groom or paw the ground instead. Splitting refers to a means of maintaining the belief that self and others are either all good or all bad. It is a somewhat immature level of defense mechanism.

34. B

35. E

36. H

37. L

38. C

39. B (Kaplan and Sadock 1988, 103). Bleuler's so-called four As consisted of associations, affect, autism, and ambivalence. He also coined the term *schizophrenia*, which means split mindedness, in reference to the theoretical schism between thought, emotion, and behavior in such patients.

40. E

41. E, 42. A, 43. D, 44. C (Wiener 1987, 228–230). With HMOs, individual or family subscribers pay an annual premium to the organization in exchange for a completely prearranged and agreed-upon group of benefits. Nonprofit insurance carriers such as Blue Cross/Blue Shield insure

about 50% of the national population and also serve as intermediaries for public programs. Medicaid is funded by the state and federal governments while Medicare is funded exclusively by the federal government. With government programs, only specified amounts are paid for services, based on customary changes for the type of service given.

45. D

46. A (Kaplan and Sadock 1988, 163–171). Stress can activate the limbic system, ultimately leading to the release of cortisol. The associated anxiety leads to increased muscle tension, heart rate, respiratory rate, and blood pressure as well as elevated serum levels of lactate, catecholamines, and cholesterol. Stress has also been linked to decreased immune function and decreased alpha waves on EEG.

47. A

48. D

49. B

50. C (Kaplan and Sadock 1988, 448–452). Anorexia nervosa commonly occurs during early to late adolescence, especially in the higher socioeconomic classes. Patients diet incessantly and, in women, amenorrhea is present. Above-average school achievement, model perfectionism, and fear of failure are also characteristic of these patients. Available evidence does not permit any conclusions about the role that heredity plays in the development of the disease. Studies have demonstrated a range of mortality rates from 5 to 18% (Kaplan and Sadock, 1988).

References

Dawson-Saunders B, Trapp R: Basic and Clinical Biostatistics. Norwalk, CT: Appleton & Lange, 1990.

Kaplan H, Sadock BJ: Clinical Psychiatry. Baltimore: Williams & Wilkins, 1988.

Simons R, Pardes H (eds): Understanding Human Behavior in Health and Illness. 2nd ed. Baltimore: Williams & Wilkins, 1981.

Wiener JM: Behavioral Science. New York: Harwal, 1987.

Pathology

1. A 33-year-old man comes to you complaining of a lump in his neck. Physical examination reveals a small thyroid nodule. The I^{131} scan that you subsequently order demonstrates a cold, 2-cm thyroid nodule. The best option of those listed below is to

A. follow this patient to see if the nodule changes in size
B. give thyroid replacement to see if the nodule shrinks
C. give TSH to see if the nodule responds by producing hormone
D. operate to remove the nodule
E. perform a fine needle aspiration biopsy of the nodule

2. In theory, the best test of thyroid function because it only measures active hormone is
   A. free thyroxine
   B. free thyroxine index (FTI)
   C. radioactive iodine uptake
   D. T3 resin uptake
   E. TRH test

3. All of the following disorders share hypertension as a common feature **except**
   A. Addison's disease
   B. adrenal medullary hyperplasia
   C. Conn's syndrome
   D. Cushing's syndrome
   E. pheochromocytoma

4. A 65-year-old African-American woman presents to you for ophthalmologic evaluation. She has had poorly controlled diabetes mellitus for 25 years. All of the following are well-recognized potential complications of her diabetes **except**
   A. glaucoma, angle-closure type
   B. neovascularization of the anterior surface of the iris
   C. retinal detachment
   D. sebaceous carcinoma of the lower eyelid
   E. snowflake cataract formation

5. Match the numbered disorders to the lettered choice that indicates the correct order from **most to least** malignant for these common skin cancers.

   1. basal cell carcinoma
   2. squamous cell carcinoma
   3. malignant melanoma

   A. 2-3-1
   B. 1-2-3
   C. 2-1-3
   D. 1-3-2
   E. 3-2-1

6. In the US, the death rate from carcinoma of the breast has been stable, but the incidence has increased. The **best** explanation for these observations is that
   A. better preventive measures are available
   B. there is an increase in smoking among women

C. the average age of the general population is increasing
D. mammography detects breast cancer at an earlier stage
E. None of these explanations is adequate to explain the observations.

7. Your patient is a 37-year-old white woman who presents with a mass in the upper outer quadrant of the left breast. Following a careful history and physical examination, you order a mammogram and fine needle aspiration of the mass. The mammographic report verifies the presence of the mass, but neither test provides a definitive diagnosis. You should now recommend
   A. a biopsy of the lesion
   B. repeat mammography in 3 to 4 months
   C. tests to detect metastatic disease
   D. that she return in a month for reexamination
   E. an ultrasound of the left breast

8. A 72-year-old woman presents with indurated plaques and nodules about the lower back and proximal thighs that have been present for about 18 months. A skin biopsy reveals mycosis fungoides cells. What histologic features are characteristic of this disorder?
   A. folded, cerebriform nuclei
   B. thickened nuclear membranes
   C. nuclear pyknosis
   D. numerous mitotic figures
   E. unusually large nucleoli

9. The most appropriate example of physiologic hyperplasia in the list below is
   A. enlargement of skeletal muscle with exercise
   B. hypertension-caused enlargement of the left ventricular wall
   C. enlargement of an organ due to edema
   D. enlargement of an organ due to increased blood flow
   E. endometrial thickening in response to stimulation by estrogen

10. During an inflammatory response, C5a mediates all of the following **except** the
    A. increase in vascular permeability
    B. influx of neutrophils
    C. upregulation of adhesion molecules on endothelial cells
    D. upregulation of adhesion molecules on neutrophils
    E. All of the above are mediated by C5a.

11. Your patient is a 51-year-old chronic alcoholic who presents with shortness of breath. On admission, he is found to have cavitary lesions in both lungs. He dies shortly after admission, and lung cultures from the autopsy grow out *Mycobacterium tuberculosis*. Which of the following would you expect to see in the sections of lung taken for microscopy?
    A. alveoli filled with lymphocytes and eosinophils
    B. alveoli filled with PMNs (segmented neutrophils)
    C. caseating granulomas with Langhans' giant cells

D. noncaseating granulomas with foreign body gaint cells
E. all of the above

12. A 72-year-old woman with a diagnosis of acute leukemia has received multiple previous blood transfusions. Her current platelet count is 8000/μl (normal = 150,000–450,000/μl). She is transfused with 8 units of platelet concentrates. Twenty minutes later, shaking chills develop and her temperature rises from 98.6 to 102.5°F. Her platelet count is still 8000/μl one hour after the transfusion. The most likely cause for this patient's reaction is
A. graft-versus-host disease
B. her antibodies directed against red blood cells in the platelet product
C. her antibodies directed against platelet proteins in the platelet product
D. her antibodies directed against white cells in the platelet product
E. a bacterial contaminant in the platelet product

13. Your attending on rounds asks you to describe the major features of non-Hodgkin's lymphoma (NHL). You should certainly include which of the following features in your response?
A. Extranodal and noncontiguous spread is rare.
B. NHL is a single disorder with several clinical and pathologic presentations.
C. NHL has a bimodal age distribution, peaking in the early 20s and also with a rising incidence after age 50.
D. Classification is based on a nodular versus diffuse pattern, coupled with cytology and B- versus T-cell immunophenotype.
E. All of these features should be included in your response.

14. A patient with cirrhosis of the liver and congestive splenomegaly has a platelet count of 60,000/mm^3 but is otherwise asymptomatic. Hemoglobin is 13.0 gm/dl and WBC is 4000/mm^3 with a normal differential. The most likely cause of the low platelet level is
A. accelerated platelet destruction
B. pooling of platelets in the spleen
C. autoimmune platelet destruction
D. disseminated intravascular coagulation
E. hematolysis malignancy

15. Of the following skin tumors, the one that is most likely to invade locally but **not** to metastasize is
A. basal cell carcinoma
B. melanoma
C. Merkel's cell carcinoma
D. mycosis fungoides
E. squamous cell carcinoma

16. A 72-year-old man presents with night sweats, weight loss, and a cavitary

lesion in the right upper lung lobe. The definitive method for identifying the etiologic agent responsible for the lung disorder is
A. acid-fast stain on lung biopsy tissue
B. acid-fast stain of sputum smears
C. lung biopsy to demonstrate granulomatous inflammation
D. culturing of acid-fast bacilli from sputum
E. strongly positive skin test

17. A 25-year-old promiscuous homosexual man presents with a 3-month history of weight loss and dry cough. *Pneumocystis carinii* pneumonia could best be diagnosed by
A. demonstrating antigen in urine
B. culturing deep tracheal secretions
C. demonstrating intranuclear inclusion bodies
D. demonstrating stainable organisms in bronchoalveolar lavage
E. demonstrating antibody in patient's serum

18. Serologic tests for syphilis such as RPR and VDRL are most likely to be negative in which stage of the disease?
A. chancre stage
B. incubation stage
C. latent stage
D. secondary stage
E. tertiary stage

19. A 65-year-old white man presents with epigastric pain of about 3 weeks' duration, and jaundice for the last 2 days. At this point, your differential diagnosis should include all of the following **except**
A. carcinoma of the head of the pancreas
B. choledochal cyst
C. stones in the common bile duct
D. viral hepatitis
E. All of these should be included.

20. Permanent liver damage can be caused by all of the following **except**
A. alpha-1-antitrypsin deficiency
B. drug reactions
C. hepatitis A virus infection
D. hereditary hemochromatosis
E. strictures of the common hepatic duct

21. The Southern blot pattern shown below represents a restriction fragment length polymorphism (RFLP) physically linked to an autosomal recessive genetic disorder. The person marked by the black square is the only one affected so far in this family. The fetus, marked "P," is calculated to be
A. affected
B. a carrier
C. an affected noncarrier

D. at 50% risk for the disorder
E. at 25% risk for the disorder

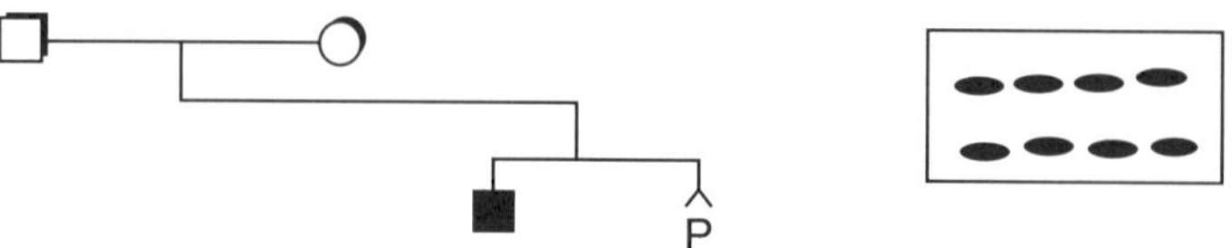

22. The incidence of neural tube defects in infants in the US is 2500 infants born per year. This incidence can be decreased if a pregnant woman does which of the following?
A. avoids smoking
B. takes folic acid
C. takes ascorbic acid
D. avoids taking thalidomide
E. takes vitamin B_{12}

Items 23–25

Select the one choice from the lettered list of bone disorders that is most closely associated with the disease described in each question. Each choice may be used once, more than once, or not at all.

A. chondrosarcoma
B. Ewing's sarcoma
C. Paget's disease of bone
D. osteochondroma (exostosis)
E. osteosarcoma

23. Common benign skeletal growth with a histologic appearance of a disorganized epiphyseal (growth plate) mechanism.
24. Tumor composed of malignant osteoblasts forming osteoid.
25. Increased osteoblastic and osteoclastic activity, resulting in weaker bones with thicker cortices and a histologic mosaic pattern either monostatic or polystatic.

26. A 25-year-old lactating woman presents with a 1-week history of swelling, redness, and tenderness in the right breast and 2 days of fever to 100°F. Physical examination confirms her findings. There is a 2-cm fluctuant mass in the upper outer quadrant. Ipsilateral axillary nodes are enlarged and tender. The most likely diagnosis is
A. breast abscess
B. infiltrating ductal carcinoma
C. inflammatory carcinoma
D. lobular carcinoma in situ
E. Paget's disease

27. Of the following, the **least** common carcinoma in the US is carcinoma arising in the
A. common bile duct
B. esophagus

C. liver
D. pancreas
E. stomach

28. All of the following factors **increase** the likelihood of developing a peptic ulcer in the gastric antrum **except**
A. cigarette smoking
B. gastrin-secreting pancreatic neoplasm
C. gastroesophageal reflux
D. infection with *Helicobacter pylori*
E. daily ingestion of aspirin for rheumatoid arthritis

29. The prognosis for patients with colorectal carcinoma is **least** dependent on which of the following factors?
A. the age of the patient
B. the extent of bowel involvement
C. histologic differentiation of the lesion
D. presence or absence of spread to lymph nodes
E. presence or absence of spread to sites beyond the limits of surgical resection

30. You have a patient whom you suspect has celiac (nontropical) sprue. You wish to perform a laboratory test to determine whether he has malabsorption. The **best** substance to measure is
A. expired hydrogen concentration after an oral lactose load
B. fecal carbohydrate
C. fecal fat
D. fecal volume
E. fecal water

31. Close and/or intermediate-range gunshot wounds may contain all of the following **except**
A. burnt gunpowder fragments
B. marginal abrasion with bullet wipe
C. muzzle imprint
D. soot
E. unburnt gunpowder fragments

32. A 65-year-old man developed a germ cell tumor of the testis. The tumor is most likely a(n)
A. embryonal carcinoma
B. Leydig cell tumor
C. mature teratoma
D. spermatocytic seminoma
E. yolk sac tumor

33. Which of the following is a correct statement regarding nodular hyperplasia of the prostate?
A. It is a precursor of prostatic carcinoma.
B. It causes urinary obstruction in 50% of cases.
C. It does not cause elevation of the prostate-specific antigen.

D. It commonly involves the peripheral zone of the prostate.
E. It is one cause of renal failure.

34. A rectal examination of an asymptomatic 55-year-old man reveals a normal-sized but indurated prostate. Prostate-specific antigen (PSA) is within normal limits. Which of the following statements is justified based on the information you have about this patient?
A. The findings are typical of prostatic hyperplasia.
B. The normal PSA definitely excludes prostatic carcinoma.
C. A urine culture would assist in diagnosis.
D. The findings are consistent with granulomatous prostatitis.
E. Prostatic biopsy will show microabscesses.

Items 35–36

Select the tumor type that is most closely associated with the statement in each question. Each lettered choice may be used once, more than once, or not at all.

A. dysgerminoma
B. endodermal sinus tumor
C. granular cell tumor
D. serous cystadenoma
E. Sertoli-Leydig cell tumor

35. This is an epithelial tumor.
36. This tumor is very radiosensitive.

37. All of the following are risk factors for squamous cell carcinoma of the cervix **except**
A. cigarette smoking
B. excess estrogen
C. certain papilloma infections
D. multiple sexual partners
E. young age at first intercourse

38. A 67-year-old man is admitted because of a stroke. On physical examination, you find that he cannot move and is blind in the left eye. He appears not to understand your questions and has great difficulty in finding the words to answer you. You suspect an occlusion in which of the following arteries?
A. left anterior choroidal
B. left internal carotid
C. left middle cerebral
D. right middle cerebral
E. right posterior cerebral

39. A 12-year-old boy developed fever, headaches, and lethargy. Lumbar puncture revealed an opening pressure of 280 mm H_2O (normal = >200 mm H_2O). The cell count was 4500/mm^3 (normal = >8 mm^3), 90% polys, sugar 25 mg/dl (normal = half of blood sugar, which was 100 mg/dl in this patient). The most likely diagnosis is

A. viral encephalitis
B. meningococcal meningitis
C. brain abscess
D. cryptococcal meningitis
E. progressive multifocal leukoencephalopathy

40. Central chromatolysis is a specific retrograde response of the neuron to injury of its
A. axon
B. cell body
C. dendrite
D. end organ
E. nucleus

41. A 70-year-old presents with crushing chest pain for the past 4 hours. Suspecting a myocardial infarct (MI), you draw blood for cardiac enzymes. Results reveal that the CP-MB band is 1.5% (normal <3%) and an LDH_1/LDH_2 ratio is 0.8 (normal <1). On these limited data, you believe the results are
A. inconsistent with a myocardial infarction
B. consistent with an MI approximately 4 hours old
C. diagnostic of an MI about 24 hours old
D. diagnostic of an MI about 48 hours old
E. due to laboratory error

42. The most common cause of sudden death following an acute myocardial infarct is
A. acute myocardial failure
B. arrhythmia
C. cardiac tamponade
D. embolism of a mural thrombus
E. rupture of a papillary muscle

43. The most common congenital condition that causes cyanotic cardiac disease is
A. aortic atresia with hypoplasia of the left ventricle
B. coarctation of the aorta
C. dextrocardia with situs inversus
D. patent foramen ovale
E. tetralogy of Fallot

44. A 10-year-old girl presents with fever, dysuria, and right flank pain. A urinary tract infection (UTI) is diagnosed. The most likely etiologic agent is
A. *Candida albicans*
B. *Escherichia coli*
C. *Pseudomonas*
D. *Staphylococcus aureus*
E. *Streptococcus pneumonia*

45. In immunologically mediated glomerulonephritis, which of the following factors contribute to glomerular injury?

A. substances secreted by macrophages
B. substances released by mesangial cells
C. substances released by platelets
D. neutrophilic enzymes
E. all of the above

46. Renal papillary necrosis in the **absence** of infection is usual in
A. analgesic abuse nephropathy
B. diabetes mellitus
C. systemic lupus erythematosus
D. urinary tract obstruction
E. Infection is typical in all of the above.

47. Inhaled particulate matter can lead to various cytokines and lysosomal enzymes being released from pulmonary macrophages. The tissue damage from such a process is most likely to result in
A. acute congestive heart failure
B. bacterial pneumonia
C. lung injury with resulting emphysema
D. pulmonary edema
E. pulmonary fibrosis leading to restrictive lung disease

48. Complications of severe bronchial asthma include
A. bronchiectasis
B. chronic bronchitis
C. cor pulmonale
D. pneumonia
E. all of the above

49. Alpha-1-antitrypsin deficiency is usually associated with which of the following conditions?
A. 28-year-old man with bullous emphysema
B. 28-year-old man with panacinar emphysema
C. 69-year-old male alcoholic with cirrhosis of the liver
D. carcinoma of the pancreas, extensively metastasized
E. hypogammaglobulinemia

50. Carcinoma in situ most commonly
A. causes no symptoms
B. causes small amounts of bleeding
C. elicits a desmoplastic response
D. metastasizes to regional lymph nodes
E. results in small, painless rashes

51. In invasion and metastases of cancer, the degradation of the extracellular matrix requires all of the following **except**
A. cathepsin
B. collagenase
C. elastase
D. glucosidase
E. lipase

52. Products of proto-oncogenes include all of the following **except**
    A. growth factors
    B. GTP-binding proteins
    C. nuclear proteins
    D. protein kinases
    E. viral capsid proteins

Explanations for Pathology Items

1. E

2. A

3. A (Robbins and Cotran 1989, 1252–1265). Addison's disease is a rare condition of adrenocortical hypofunction, with many potential etiologies. It is characterized by the insidious onset of fatigue, weakness, nausea, anorexia, hypoglycemia, hyperpigmentation, and hypotension. It is the mineralocorticoid loss that is responsible for the hypotension, secondary to renal sodium wasting, potassium retention, and resultant severe dehydration. The other choices all manifest hypertension, along with other unique characteristic signs and symptoms.

4. D

5. E

6. D

7. A (Robbins and Cotran 1989, 1192–1201). The information obtained via history, physical exam, and mammogram was sufficient to warrant further investigation, particularly in light of the fact that the best prognosis in breast cancer occurs in cases of early identification, when the mass is less than 2.0 cm and no nodal metastases have occurred. Fine needle aspiration has many advantages including lower cost and better patient tolerance; however, limitations include lack of normal histologic tissue to compare and the possiblity of erroneous sampling, missing diagnostic material. The next best choice is biopsy. Waiting even 1 month may be too late. Ultrasound is not used in the evaluation of breast masses.

8. A (Robbins and Cotran 1989, 716–718, 1293–1294). Mycosis fungoides (MF) is an uncommon cutaneous T-cell lymphoma, with three stages of skin manifestations: *erythremia, plagues (eczema-like),* and *tumors.* The malignant cells are predominantly arranged as a band in the upper dermis, and as clusters extending into the epidermis. The characteristic cell is a CD4 helper, T cell. It has a large, markedly irregular nucleus, commonly referred to as cerebriform or "serpentine." The nuclear rim is generally not thickened and the nucleolus, though prominent, is not particularly large or eosinophilic. Nuclear pyknosis and frequent mitoses do occur, but are not unique to MF. When it involves skin, nodes, and

peripheral blood, it is known as Sézary syndrome (the leukemic phase of mycoses fungoides).

9. E

10. C (Robbins and Cotran 1989, 45–46, 53–54). C5a is a cleavage product formed from the complement protein C5, via both the classic and alternate complement pathways. It has a number of functional properties: increased vascular permeability (anaphylatoxin); chemotaxis for neutrophils, eosinophils, and macrophages; and upregulation of adhesion molecules on leukocytes. Upregulation of adhesion molecules on endothelial cells is induced by some inflammatory mediators such as interleukin-1.

11. C (Robbins and Cotran 1989, 64–65, 374–380). *Mycobacterium tuberculosis* is a slender, acid-fast slow-growing bacillus. In tissue sections, it usually induces a characteristic caseating granuloma that is composed of a rim of epithelioid histocytes, fibroblasts, lymphocytes, and occasional Langhans' giant cells, with a central area of coagulative and liquefaction (caseous) necrosis. In some immunocompromised patients, especially those with AIDS, well-formed granulomas may not occur, and therefore reliance on cultures or Gram's stains, or both, to detect the organism is critical. This is one of the most important bacterial pathogens, with a worldwide distribution. It flourishes in crowded conditions, and in malnourished and debilitated individuals. The incidence of drug resistance (frequently multidrug resistance) has risen dramatically, so that this is now also of increasingly significant concern for immunocompromised patients and health care workers.

12. D

13. D (Robbins and Cotran 1989, 708–722). Non-Hodgkin's lymphoma (NHL) encompasses a spectrum of lymphomas with numerous, frequently confusing forms. These differ in cell of origin; occurrences in various age groups, races, sexes, and geographic locations; response to treatment; and prognosis. NHL has frequent involvement of multiple peripheral lymph nodes, shows noncontiguous spread, and frequently involves Waldeyer's ring, mesenteric nodes, and extranodal spread. In contrast, Hodgkin's disease encompasses four main subclasses, unique in the presence of Reed-Sternberg or Hodgkin's malignant cells. It characteristically shows a bimodal age distribution (20 and 50), is usually localized to a single axial group of lymph nodes, shows contiguous spread, and rarely shows involvement of Waldeyer's ring, mesenteric nodes, or extranodal spread.

14. B (Robbins and Cotran 1989, 749, 941–957). Cirrhosis of the liver is the most common cause of portal hypertension that manifests as ascites, portosystemic shunts (for example, esophageal varices), occasional hepatic encephalopathy, and splenomegaly, which can be massive. Splenomegaly may in turn cause sequestration of red and white blood cells, as well as platelets (most common), resulting in clinically signifi-

cant decreases in any one or a combination of these. Choices A, C, and D are unlikely to occur in a classic cirrhotic with no other abnormalities. A hematologic malignancy would likely manifest abnormalities in the hemoglobin or WBCs or both, as well as platelets.

15. A (Robbins and Cotran 1989, 248, 1286–1290). Most malignant tumors metastasize; indeed, for some tumors, evidence of metastasis is critical to classify the tumor as malignant, because they fail to demonstrate characteristic malignant cellular features and may not show local invasion. Exceptions to this include basal cell carcinoma of the skin and most of the glial neoplasms of the central nervous system. The reason for this is not known. The other dermatologic malignancies listed do metastasize to variable degrees.

16. D (Robbins and Cotran 1989, 374–380; see question 11). The definitive method for identifying *any culturable* infectious agent is microbiologic. Special stains are orders of magnitude *less* sensitive, and thus may not detect organisms in low numbers. In addition, the tissue sections selected for examination may fail to contain the organisms. Granulomatous inflammation can occur in a variety of infectious as well as noninfectious conditions, and thus is not specific enough to use for determining the appropriate treatment modality. In immunocompromised individuals (such as those with AIDS), skin tests may not work and granulomas may not form, and thus, depending on them for diagnosis is not acceptable.

17. D (Robbins and Cotran 1989, 401–402, 783–784). *Pneumocystis carinii* (PC) is an organism that appears closely related to fungi. It is ubiquitous in distribution, and represents an opportunistic agent, causing pulmonary infiltrates and infections in the course of the disease. The alveolar spaces (not trachea or bronchi) contain foamy pale-pink material in which the organism resides. The best mode of diagnosis is a bronchoalveolar lavage or lung biopsy stained with a silver stain to demonstrate the cup-like trophozoite cysts. Currently, there are no serologic (antigen/antibody) or culture methods to diagnose PC, although this represents an area of ongoing research.

18. B

19. B

20. C (Robbins and Cotran 1989, 924–940). Hepatitis A is caused by a small, nonenveloped, single-stranded RNA virus. Transmission is by the oral-fecal route. Military areas, prisons, and daycare settings all are situations where outbreaks can occur. It is a relatively benign, self-limiting disease, with rare (0.1%) occurrences of fatal fulminant hepatitis. There are no chronic or carrier forms of this disease, and permanent liver damage does not occur, as it would with any of the other viral forms or drug hepatitis. The hereditary diseases and the stricture of the ducts all have cirrhosis as an endpoint.

21. D

22. B

23. D

24. E

25. C

26. A (Robbins and Cotran 1989, 1182–1201). Acute mastitis is a common occurrence in the early weeks of lactation and nursing, when dryness and fissures can occur in the nipples. The potential for infection is present, with common organisms including staphylococci and streptococci. Symptoms include pain, swelling, redness, warmth, axillary lymphadenopathy, fever, and malaise. This may go on to abscess formation, which can be multicentric. If untreated, dense fibrosis can occur, with mass formation and skin puckering, mimicking cancer. Carcinoma in situ generally does not form a palpable mass, and while the other cancers do present as notable lesions, in general all are nontender and do not demonstrate systemic symptoms.

27. A

28. C (Robbins and Cotran 1989, 848–854). Ninety-eight to ninety-nine percent of peptic ulcer disease occurs in the duodenum or stomach in a 4 : 1 ratio; however, it can occur in any part of the GI tract exposed to gastric acids. The primary alteration responsible in the gastric type is altered resistance of the mucosa to acids (breakdown of the mucosal barrier) in the paradoxical face of common achlorhydria. Other factors include elderly, female, smoking, aspirin or other nonsteroidal antiinflammatory drug (NSAID) use, and *Helicobacter* (old *Campylobacter*) *pylori* infection, all of which alter the mucosal barrier. An uncommon cause is the gastrin-secreting neoplasm (gastrinoma) of Zollinger-Ellison syndrome. Gastroesophageal reflux is associated with reflux *esophagitis*, of which Barrett's is a potentially premalignant form.

29. A

30. C (Robbins and Cotran 1989, 876–879). Malabsorption syndromes include a diverse group of diseases with unique etiologies (some unknown) and histologies. All, however, demonstrate a similar constellation of signs and symptoms that can be very severe and life threatening. Bulky, greasy, and/or frothy stools are a hallmark and the fat content can be assessed to diagnose malabsorption and its severity. One of the more common forms is celiac sprue, also known as gluten-sensitive or nontropical sprue. It is believed to be due to a hypersensitivity reaction to the gliadin protein within gluten, which is found in wheat, barley, and rye. In most cases, the only way to determine which form of malabsorption is present is to do a biopsy, which is important because each type has a different treat-

ment and prognosis. Hydrogen content, or the "hydrogen breath test," is used in assessing lactate deficiency and several other malabsorption problems, but has not been found useful in diagnosis of sprue.

31. C

32. D

33. E (Robbins and Cotran 1989, 1118–1121). Nodular hyperplasia, previously known as benign prostatic hyperplasia, involves the growth of periurethral (central) nodules of benign fibromuscular and glandular tissue. It is very common in men over the age of 50 and is *not* a premalignant condition. Clinically significant obstruction requiring surgery occurs in 5 to 10% of cases. If not corrected, complications of pyelonephritis, hydronephritis, and eventual renal failure can occur. Prostatic-specific antigen, or PSA, can be elevated in nodular hyperplasia, prostatic manipulation, inflammatory conditions, and carcinoma, although the higher the elevation, the more likely that it is due to cancer. Ultrasound-guided biopsies of *hypo*echoic areas within the prostate, regardless of its size, can help to pick out malignant lesions, which *can occur simultaneously* with nodular hyperplasia.

34. D

35. D

36. A

37. B (Robbins and Cotran 1989, 275–277, 1142–1145, 1154). The most significant risk factors for cervical carcinoma include early age at first sexual intercourse, multiple sexual partners, and any partner with a *previous* partner who experienced cervical carcinoma, or who has genital condylomas. The common denominator here is exposure to human papilloma virus (HPV). This causes condyloma acuminatum (subtypes 6 and 11), and other warts. It has been detected in 90 to 95% of all cervical squamous cell carcinomas (subtypes 16 and 18) and is strongly suspected to be an oncogenic agent, making cervical squamous carcinoma a sexually transmitted disease. In numerous studies, cigarette smoking has also been implicated, probably relating to its increased occurrence among persons who are more likely to be engaging in the above-listed risk behaviors. Estrogen excess is a risk factor for endometrial and breast cancer.

38. B

39. B

40. A (Robbins and Cotran 1989, 1386–1387). Central chromatolysis, also known as axonal reaction, occurs if an axon is cut. This disrupts the axonal flow of neuronal cytoplasm, which then collects in the cell body. The result is distention and peripheral displacement of the nucleus and

Nissl substance (free ribosomes). The residual structure is pale staining (chromatolysis). Nuclear damage results in cell death. Damage to the other listed structures has variable effects, depending on the extent and etiology of the damage.

41. B (Robbins and Cotran 1989, 604–614). Serum enzyme levels are the traditional method of diagnosis in a possible myocardial infarction (MI), in conjunction with clinical findings and ECG changes. The first enzyme to elevate and decline is the CK-MB isoenzyme of creatinine kinase. This is detectable approximately 4 to 8 hours after the event, and returns to normal at 3 to 4 days. LDH elevates at about 24 hours and remains elevated for up to 2 weeks. The LDH isoenzyme change that is diagnostic for an MI occurs when the LDH_1 becomes greater than the LDH_2, which is known as the "LD flip." In this situation, the enzymes are normal; thus, the correct interpretation is that either no MI occurred or that it occurred less than 4 hours previously. A number of newer, nonenzymatic techniques to diagnose MI are being developed, so that earlier and more certain detection will soon be possible.

42. B

43. E

44. B (Robbins and Cotran 1989, 345–346, 1052–1053). Urinary tract infections include both cystitis (bladder) and pyelonephritis (kidney) infections. These are most common among women aged 15 to 40, which is thought to be due to factors such as shorter urethras, lack of prostatic fluid (which has antibacterial properties), hormonal changes, and urethral trauma during intercourse. Eighty-five percent are caused by gram-negative bacilli, with *E. coli* the most common, but they can be caused by virtually any bacteria or fungus, with the fungal infections more often occurring in debilitated patients, with biliary tract obstructions or congenital abnormalities.

45. E

46. A

47. E

48. E

49. B

50. A (Robbins and Cotran 1989, 243, 246, 1142). Some cancers evolve from a preinvasive lesion known as *carcinoma in situ* (CIS) or intraepithelial neoplasia. This generally occurs in surface epithelial tumors, such as cervical, rectal, bronchial, or esophageal. It represents a state *prior to* a membrane breach, and thus does not involve vascular, lymphatic, or perineural invasion. The classic example is that of cervical squamous CIS, which can evolve over years or, in rare circumstances,

recede without producing any symptoms or masses. Once bleeding is noted, micro or frank invasion is likely. Metastasis requires breach of lymphatics or vasculature, which has not yet occurred in CIS, and a desmoplastic reaction only occurs in invasive tumors.

51. E

52. E

Reference

Robbins SL, Cotran RS: Pathologic Basis of Disease. 4th ed. Philadelphia: Saunders, 1989.

Microbiology

1. Prokaryotic cells have all of the following features **except** that they
   A. have no organelles or histones
   B. have cells walls of peptidoglycan
   C. can be diploid or haploid
   D. have short-lived mRNA
   E. have coupled transcription and translation

2. You are treating a 32-year-old female immunocompromised patient who has had intermittent headaches, dizziness, and mental confusion that have gradually increased in severity. A CSF sample is cultured with negative India ink stain, revealing encapsulated yeast cells. Of the following, the most likely etiologic agent is
   A. blastomycosis
   B. coccidioidomycosis
   C. histoplasmosis
   D. cryptococcosis
   E. candidiasis

3. *Aspergillus* species cause a variety of human diseases when conidia are inhaled. Once established, the fungi can produce
   A. asthma
   B. endocarditis
   C. a fungus ball
   D. noninvasive bronchitis
   E. all of the above

4. A 7-year-old boy is brought to the ER complaining of abdominal pain for about 3 days. There is no diarrhea, but he has a low-grade fever. As the mother indicates that her 10-year-old daughter was recently treated for "some kind of worms," you obtain a fecal sample, which reveals numerous elliptically shaped eggs with a rough, albumin-like coat over

a thin, chitinous shell. You prescribe mebendazole for this infection, whose etiologic agent is
A. *Ascaris lumbricoides*
B. *Enterobius vermicularis*
C. *Toxocara canis*
D. *Trichuris trichiura*
E. *Trichinella spiralis*

5. In working up a 2-year-old child for suspected meningitis, CSF testing helps you differentiate between viral and bacterial forms. True statements about viral meningitis include all of the following **except**
A. enteroviruses and mumps are primary causes
B. infections commonly occur in late winter and early spring
C. it rarely occurs in patients over age 40
D. signs and symptoms become apparent gradually
E. CSF leukocyte counts in excess of 1000 are characteristic

6. Regarding urinary tract infections, all of the following are correct statements **except**
A. females are 10 times more likely than males to contract UTIs
B. the risk of UTI in females is unrelated to age
C. diabetes significantly increases the risk of UTIs
D. kidney stones can increase the risk of UTIs
E. *E. coli* accounts for most cases of UTI

7. A 42-year-old HIV-positive man presents in the ER with tachypnea, nasal flaring, a fever of 40°C, and shaking chills. Chest auscultation is unremarkable. A chest x-ray reveals diffuse granular infiltrates in both lungs. The most likely etiologic agent is
A. adenovirus type 4
B. *Streptococcus pneumoniae*
C. *Klebsiella pneumoniae*
D. *Legionella pneumophila*
E. *Pneumocystis carinii*

Items 8–12

Select the organism that is most closely associated with each statement. Each choice may be used once, more than once, or not at all.

A. *Actinomyces israelii*
B. *Erysipelothrix rhusiopathiae*
C. *Legionella pneumophila*
D. *Listeria monocytogenes*
E. *Mycoplasma pneumoniae*
F. *Nocardia asteroides*
G. *Ureaplasma urealyticum*
H. *Mycoplasma hominis*
I. *Corynebacterium diphtheriae*

8. Forms a pseudomembrane in the oropharynx.
9. Causes a severe pneumonia with a mortality rate as high as 15–20%.

10. Is associated with draining sinus tracts.
11. Can produce postabortion or postpartum fevers.
12. Produces an infection often referred to as walking pneumonia.

13. A 17-year-old member of a Midwestern water polo team presents in your office with an ulcerated lesion on the back of the left hand. He states that he has a vague memory of scraping his hand on the edge of the pool about 10 days ago. The most likely etiologic agent is
    A. *Mycobacterium kansasii*
    B. *Mycobacterium marinum*
    C. *Mycobacterium intracellulare*
    D. *Mycobacterium scrufulaceum*
    E. *Mycobacterium ulcerans*

14. All of the following statements about whooping cough are correct **except**
    A. it is most infectious in the paroxysmal coughing stage
    B. it is caused by *Bordetella pertussis*
    C. the etiologic agent is an obligate human parasite
    D. symptoms are mostly due to the host's response to toxins
    E. a member of the same genus causes kennel cough in puppies

15. Three cases of salmonella poisoning are reported in a local newspaper the day following a large company picnic. Public health workers investigate to determine the source of the contamination. The most likely source, given the following menu items that were consumed by all of the victims, is
    A. milk
    B. fried chicken
    C. jello salad
    D. fried catfish
    E. popsicles

Items 16–18

For each of the following items, match the organism to the statement with which it is most closely associated. Each choice may be used once, more than once, or not at all.

A. *Bacillus anthracis*
B. *Clostridium perfringens*
C. short-duration gastroenteritis
D. *Clostridium difficile*
E. *Bacillus subtilis*

16. Can cause a disorder known as woolsorter's disease.
17. Fried rice is a common source.
18. It is one etiologic agent in gas gangrene.

19. Viruses share all of the following features **except**
    A. they are universally obligate intracellular parasites
    B. their genomes are inside a protective shell

C. each contains only one type of nucleic acid
D. there is no reliable method for directly detecting them
E. they infect virtually all natural organisms

Items 20–23

Match the descriptions of viral replication patterns to the appropriate virus group. Each lettered choice may be used once, more than once, or not at all.

A. poliovirus
B. rhabdovirus
C. herpesviruses
D. poxviruses
E. retroviruses

20. A unique feature makes it impossible to obtain infectious RNA from this group.
21. Uses a double-stranded DNA intermediate.
22. The viral RNA is translated into a single giant polypeptide of 200,000 to 300,000 molecular weight.
23. The virus itself contains an RNA polymerase.

Items 24–27

Match each description of a chemical inhibitor to the appropriate term. Each lettered choice may be used once, more than once, or not at all.

A. adenosine arabinoside (ara-A)
B. amantadine
C. dideoxynucleoside (e.g., AZT)
D. ribavirin (Virazole)
E. rifampin

24. Highly toxic inhibitor of reverse transcriptase in retroviruses.
25. Antiviral activity against influenza A viruses.
26. FDA-approved for treatment of acquired immunodeficiency syndrome.
27. An analogue used to treat human infections caused by herpes viruses, it inhibits viral DNA polymerase.

28. All of the following are routine methods for diagnosing viral infections **except**
    A. propagation in cell cultures or by animal inoculation
    B. assessment of immune cell function
    C. serologic typing
    D. immunofluorescence
    E. recognition of clinical presentation pattern

29. All of the following are correct characteristics of Orthomyxoviridae infections **except**
    A. antigenic variation is due to surface spike glycoproteins
    B. major antigenic shifts have occurred four times since 1933

C. they may cause epidemic illnesses
D. they occur primarily during the summer
E. spread is from person to person by aerosolization

Items 30–33

Each of the following statements describes a specific viral disease. Match each statement to the proper etiologic agent. Each lettered choice may be used once, more than once, or not at all.

A. Coxsackie virus A
B. Epstein-Barr virus
C. hepatitis B virus
D. influenza virus
E. poliovirus
F. respiratory syncytial virus
G. rhabdovirus
H. rotavirus
I. rubella virus
J. smallpox virus
K. varicella-zoster virus

30. Affects lymphoid tissue, causing fever, fatigue, and sore throat; its most common disease form affects mainly middle- and upper-class persons aged 16 to 20.
31. Following a 14- to 16-day incubation, fever develops, followed by a papular rash of the skin and mucous membranes.
32. Classified as a togavirus, this virus can damage all germ layers in a fetus.
33. This virus is associated with severe infantile gastroenteritis.

34. All of the following statements are correct characterizations of innate (nonspecific) immunity factors **except**
A. mechanical barriers inhibit attachment of infectious agents
B. tears contain a component that lyses bacterial cell walls
C. an increase in corticosteroids enhances the inflammatory response
D. a high oxygen tension inhibits the growth of anaerobes in the lungs
E. the acid pH of most bodily secretions helps prevent colonization

35. Adaptive immunity includes all of the following features **except**
A. immunologic memory
B. induction
C. pinocytosis
D. self-recognition
E. specificity

Items 36–38

Match each definitional statement to the most closely associated term. Each lettered choice may be used once, more than once, or not at all.

A. affinity
B. antigenicity
C. avidity
D. coulombic forces
E. van der Waal's forces

36. The strength of the interaction between multivalent antigens and the population that they have induced.
37. The property of a substance that enables it to react with the specific lymphocyte that caused it to be produced.
38. Patterns of complementary electrical charge on molecules that tend to hold the molecules together.

39. Which of the following diseases is characterized by hypoplasia of the face, thymus, and parotid glands, and nearly normal levels of immunoglobulins, but a markedly decreased number of T cells?
A. ataxia-telangiectasia
B. Bruton's agammaglobulinemia
C. Chédiak-Higashi syndrome
D. Di George's syndrome
E. Wiskott-Aldrich syndrome

40. All of the following statements regarding the humoral immune response are correct **except**
A. the development of full immunocompetence takes several years
B. IgM synthesis begins before birth
C. IgG in colostrum provides local immunity in an infant's upper respiratory and GI tracts
D. IgG is acquired from the mother and is the major fetal antibody
E. very premature infants tend to have extremely low levels of all immunoglobulins

41. Which statement correctly defines the term **tolerance**?
A. The ability to enhance or augment an immune response.
B. A congenital defect that reduces a large portion of the immune response.
C. The suppression of an autoimmune response.
D. The absence of an immune response to a substrate that has all the features necessary for antigenicity.
E. The absence of a specific immune response.

Items 42–45

Match each description of immunization methods for specific diseases to the appropriate term. Each lettered choice may be used once, more than once, or not at all.

A. live, attenuated virus vaccine
B. killed (inactivated) vaccine
C. toxoid

D. Dead bacterial vaccine
E. attenuated bacterial vaccine

42. mumps vaccine
43. oral polio (Sabin) vaccine
44. pertussis vaccine
45. diphtheria vaccine

46. You are treating a 37-year-old female patient who complains of limb pain and fatigue for the past year. She was recently treated for a fractured tibia and was treated for a similar injury on the left about 11 months ago. Suspicious, you order a complete blood panel, which reveals the presence of paraprotein (M component) in addition to normochromic, normocytic anemia. She also demonstrates an abnormally high level of IgG. On reading these results, you are certain that the patient suffers from
    A. amyloidosis
    B. chronic granulomatous disease
    C. multiple myeloma
    D. rheumatoid arthritis
    E. Waldenström's macroglobulinemia

Items 47–49

Match each disease depiction to the autoimmune disorder that it most closely describes. Each lettered choice may be used once, more than once, or not at all.

A. acute disseminated encephalomyelitis
B. Guillain-Barré syndrome
C. multiple sclerosis
D. myasthenia gravis
E. systemic lupus erythematosus

47. A postinfectious disease with progressive weakness of the extremites and respiratory muscles. Return of function is typically seen in 6 to 10 months.
48. Chronic muscle weakness and fatigue resulting from depletion of acetylcholine receptors at the myoneural junction.
49. A chronic, multi-organ disorder that most frequently affects young women of childbearing age.

50. All of the following statements regarding transplantation are correct **except**
    A. a platelet transfusion is an example of an allograft
    B. graft-versus-host reactions are an expression of B-cell function
    C. in humans, the major histocompatibility complex resides on the short arm of chromosome 6
    D. isografts can survive indefinitely
    E. kidneys are the most frequently transplanted organs

Explanations for Microbiology Items

1. C (Joklik et al. 1992, 8). Living organisms produce two types of cells: prokaryotic and eukaryotic. Prokaryotic cells have no membrane-bound organelles such as Golgi bodies and lysosomes. They do not have histones binding their DNA, as do eukaryotic cells. Prokaryotic cells contain a single, circular, double-stranded DNA molecule and are considered haploid. Because they are not compartmentalized, translation of proteins will begin before transcription of the messenger RNA is complete. The short-lived mRNA of prokaryotes is a form of regulation for the protein composition of the cell. With the exception of mycoplasmas (which do not contain cell walls), all prokaryotes produce a cell wall containing peptidoglycan.

2. D

3. E

4. A (Berkow and Fletcher 1987, 214–225). *Ascaris lumbricoides,* commonly known as the giant intestinal roundworm, has the highest infection rates in humans by intestinal nematodes. All these parasitic infections can cause a low-grade fever; however, only *Trichuris trichiura* (whipworm), *Enterobius vermicularis* (pinworm), and *Ascaris lumbricoides* can cause abdominal pain. The key diagnostic feature is the identification of the eggs in a stool sample. *Trichinella spiralis* may cause gastrointestinal problems within the first few days of infection, but symptoms often go unnoticed by the patient.

5. E

6. B (Berkow and Fletcher 1987, 1610–1619). *Escherichia coli* accounts for about 85% of uncomplicated urinary tract infections (UTIs). Females are 10 times more likely than males to contract UTIs. The prevalence of UTIs in females is about 1% between infancy and adolescence, rising to 2 to 3% between age 20 and 60 years, then 10 to 20% for older women. Obstruction by kidney stones increases the risk of UTIs by causing stasis, allowing the growth of invading bacteria. Adults with diabetes mellitus have a higher incidence of UTIs because of more frequent urination and greater susceptibility to tissue invasion.

7. E (Joklik et al. 1992, 1184–1185). *Pneumocystis carinii* is an opportunistic pathogen in immunocompromised individuals. The mode of transmission appears to be the inhalation of cysts, containing up to eight pear-shaped sporozoites. *Pneumocystis carinii* is the cause of about 60% of deaths in patients with AIDS. The onset of infection is abrupt. Acute cases present with fever and tachypnea; after one week, a flaring of the nasal alae and cyanosis occur. Radiographs will show a diffuse bilateral alveolar disease with interstitial plasma cell pneumonitis, with a ground-glass appearance. Definitive diagnosis is demonstrated by identifying the organism using special stains in samples taken by needle biopsy, bronchial brushing or lavage (Joklik et al. 1992).

8. I (Brooks et al. 1991, 189). *Corynebacterium diphtheriae* infects the epithelium in the upper respiratory tract. The toxin is absorbed into the mucous membrane. The resulting necrotic epithelium becomes embedded in exuding fibrin with red and white blood cells forming a pseudomembrane. This grayish pseudomembrane commonly covers the tonsils, pharynx, or larynx, and any attempt to remove the pseudomembrane exposes and tears the capillaries, resulting in bleeding.

9. C

10. A

11. H (Brooks et al. 1991, 268–269). *Mycoplasma hominis* has been associated with postpartum and postabortion fevers. It has been found with other bacteria in uterine tube infections, and is associated with pelvic inflammatory disease. Treatment by tetracycline or erythromycin suppress the organism.

12. E (Brooks et al. 1991, 270). *Mycoplasma pneumoniae* is the most common pathogen for lung infections among children and young adults from 5 to 35 years old. The organism destroys the ciliated epithelial cells of the respiratory tract mucosa. An incubation period of 1 to 3 weeks is followed by initial symptoms that resemble influenza. The generally mild disease progresses gradually for 1 to 2 weeks, after which there is spontaneous recovery. Because the disease has a mild progression, it is sometimes referred to as walking pneumonia.

13. B (Berkow and Fletcher 1987, 126). *Mycobacterium marinum* and *M. ulcerans* are normally found in water, grow best at low temperature (31°C), and can produce superficial skin lesions in humans. *M. marinum* causes "swimming pool granulomas," which usually heal spontaneously. *M. ulcerans* causes an indolent, progressive, cutaneous and subcutaneous ulceration seen only in Africa and Australia. *M. kansasii, M. intracellulare*, and *M. scrufulaceum* cause chronic pulmonary disease that is very similar to tuberculosis.

14. A (Brooks et al. 1991, 239–241). *Bordetella pertussis*, the causative agent of whooping cough, is transmitted through the respiratory route from early cases and possibly by carriers. There is no vector for this obligate human parasite; the bacterium survives for only brief periods outside the human host. The organism interferes with ciliary action as it multiplies on the epithelial surface of the trachea and bronchi. Pertussis toxin is released, irritating the cells, causing coughing and marked lymphocytosis. After an incubation period of 2 weeks, the "catarrhal" stage begins, which is the most infectious stage. Mild coughing and sneezing develop, releasing large numbers of organisms sprayed in the droplets. During the "paroxysmal" stage, the patient develops the characteristic explosive cough with a "whoop" on inhalation. A member of the same genus, *Bordetella bronchiseptica*, causes kennel cough in dogs.

15. B

16. A

17. C

18. B

19. D

20. B (Brooks et al. 1991, 539). Rhabdoviruses are enveloped, bullet-shaped viruses that contain a single-stranded, negative-sense RNA. Since the RNA does not serve as a messenger, it is not infectious. The virions contain an RNA-dependent RNA polymerase so that, upon infection of the cell, the virus transcribes its own messenger RNA. One well-known member is the rabies virus.

21. E (Brooks et al. 1991, 557–558). Retroviruses are single-stranded RNA viruses that must go through a double-stranded DNA intermediate before viral expression. On infection of a cell, retroviruses carry with them a reverse transcriptase enzyme that will transcribe a double-stranded DNA copy of the virus's RNA. This DNA is integrated into the host DNA, where it serves as a template for host RNA polymerase.

22. A (Joklik et al. 1992, 813–815). Poliovirus is a single-stranded positive-sense RNA virus. After the virus infects the cell and is uncoated, the poliovirus RNA serves as a messenger RNA and translates into one large polypeptide between 200,000 and 300,000 molecular weight. The polypeptide is specifically cleaved by viral proteases.

23. D (Brooks et al. 1991, 441). Poxviruses are the largest and most complex viruses. They are enveloped virions that contain a double-stranded DNA genome. The virion contains many enzymes, including RNA polymerase, and therefore its own transcriptional system can synthesize, polyadenylate, cap, and methylate viral messenger RNA.

24. E (Dulbecco and Ginsberg 1988, 114–115). Rifampin and its derivatives are moderate to strong inhibitors of reverse transcriptase activity in retroviruses. However, the dosage necessary to treat patients effectively would be highly toxic to the patient because rifampin also inhibits cellular DNA polymerase activity at these high doses.

25. B (Brooks et al. 1991, 401). Amantadine is a synthetic amine that specifically inhibits influenza A viruses by interfering with viral penetration into the host cell and blocking viral uncoating. When administered prophylactically, amantadine has a significant protective effect in humans against influenza A but not against influenza B or other viruses.

26. C (Brooks et al. 1991, 398). Dideoxynucleosides, specifically 3-azido-3-deoxythymidine (AZT), are synthetic thymidine analogues that inhibit DNA synthesis. However, HIV's reverse transcriptase enzyme is

100 times more sensitive to this analogue than cellular DNA polymerase, thereby blocking proviral synthesis. Unfortunately, as with all dideoxynucleosides, this drug causes toxic side effects including bone marrow suppression, and patients must therefore be closely monitored.

27. A (Brooks et al. 1991, 399). Adenosine arabinoside (ara-A) is a purine analogue that blocks viral DNA synthesis by inhibiting viral-specific DNA polymerase. Ara-A has been used topically to treat corneal lesions due to herpes simplex virus. With varicella-zoster infections (chickenpox), new lesion formation and duration of fever have been shown to decrease after ara-A treatment. Ara-A is relatively nontoxic but may cause nausea and phlebitis.

28. B

29. D

30. B

31. K

32. I

33. H

34. C

35. C (Brooks et al. 1991, 105–108). Adaptive or acquired immunity is the immunologic response to foreign antigens that induces lymphocytes to proliferate. On first exposure to an antigen or subsequent re-exposure, there is an inductive phase during which time lymphocytes proliferate into antibody-secreting plasma cells or reactive T cells. Immunologic memory is the long-term resistance after initial contact with a foreign antigen. The contact may be from a clinical or subclinical infection, immunization, exposure to microbial products, or transplantation of foreign cells. The specificity of the immune system is evidenced by its reacting only with homologous antigens and by its ability to discriminate self-antigens from foreign antigens. Pinocytosis is an innate characteristic of cells used to internalize fluids and solutes.

36. C

37. B

38. D

39. D (Berkow and Fletcher 1987, 284). Di George's syndrome is a congenital immunodeficiency characterized by the absence or hypoplasia of the thymus and parathyroid gland. Immunologically, patients have a normal to near normal B-cell immunity but a partial or complete T-cell deficiency. Affected infants have low-set ears, midline facial clefts, a

shortened philtrum, a small receding mandible, and hypertelorism. The degree of immunodeficiency varies from patient to patient and sometimes T-cell function improves spontaneously. Treatment consists of fetal thymic transplants or bone marrow transplantation.

40. C

41. E

42. A (Brooks et al. 1991, 525–527). A live attentuated mumps virus vaccine was licensed in 1967, resulting in a reduction of mumps cases from 200,000 cases in 1967 to 300 cases in 1985. Replication initially occurs in the epithelial cells of the nasal or upper respiratory tract. The virus then disseminates to the salivary glands and other major organs. Incubation is about 18 days, with virus being shed 6 days to one week after salivary swelling. An attenuated live vaccine is given as a single dose subcutaneously. Antibodies are detectable in 95% of vaccinees, and the antibody persists for at least 10 years. The vaccine may be given in monovalent form or in combination with rubella (MR) or measles and rubella (MMR).

43. A (Brooks et al. 1991, 471–473). Poliomyelitis is an infectious viral disease that, in its most serious form, affects the central nervous system. The virus enters the mouth and replicates in the intestine and oropharynx. The virus is excreted in the stools for several weeks. Antibodies to the virus appear early in the disease; however, a small percentage of cases progress to paralytic poliomyelitis. Before vaccines were developed, 21,000 cases were seen in the US per year. Currently, the disease has almost vanished in industrialized countries. Two vaccines were developed: The oral polio (Sabin) vaccine is a live attenuated virus that thereby stimulates IgG and IgM as well as IgA in the intestine. The other vaccine is the killed virus (Salk) vaccine, which must be given four times over a 1- to 2-year period.

44. D (Brooks et al. 1991, 239–241). The pertussis vaccine is given three times during the first year of life, usually in combination with toxoids of diphtheria and tetanus (DTP). The pertussis component is a killed crude suspension of bacteria that is an effective immunogen but with variable vaccine quality and acceptance. Inadequate active immunization of all infants is the major reason that whooping cough is not under control. Most cases occur in children under age 5 and most deaths occur in infants less than 1 year old.

45. C (Brooks et al. 1991, 188–191). *Corynebacterium diphtheriae* is the causative agent for diphtheria. This gram-positive club-shaped rod grows on the mucous membrane of the upper respiratory tract or in minor skin wounds. Strains of *C. diphtheriae* carry a temperate bacteriophage with a structural gene for a toxin. The toxin is made of two fragments; fragment B has no activity except to carry fragment A into the cell, where fragment A inhibits protein synthesis. The diphtheria vaccine is a toxoid, whose toxicity has been destroyed by a low concentration of formaldehyde.

46. C

47. B (Berkow and Fletcher 1987, 1446). Guillain-Barré syndrome is an acute, rapidly progressive form of polyneuropathy characterized by a weakness of extremities and respiratory muscles that occurrs about 5 days to 3 weeks after either an infectious disorder, surgery, or immunization. The etiology is unknown. Respiratory paralysis and the autonomic defects may be life threatening. Considerable improvement over a period of a month is usual; however, 30% of adults may have residual weakness at 3 years.

48. D (Berkow and Fletcher 1987, 1449). Myasthenia gravis is a disease caused by an autoimmune attack on the acetylcholine receptor of the postsynaptic neuromuscular junction. The antibody attack results in a loss of acetylcholine receptors causing chronic muscle fatigue. The disease commonly presents between 20 to 40 years of age, predominantly affecting women. The condition is rare and symptoms may be vague; therefore, diagnosis can be missed. Diagnosis is confirmed by improvement with anticholinesterase drugs.

49. E (Berkow and Fletcher 1987, 1274–1277). Systemic lupus erythematosus is an autoimmune disease in which the patient produces antinuclear antibodies. A chronic inflammatory connective tissue disorder occurs predominantly in young women of childbearing age. Women account for 90% of cases. Diagnosis is made when the patient has a febrile disease with an erythematous skin rash, leukopenia, polyarthritis, evidence of renal disease, and hyperglobulinemia with anti-DNA antibodies. Prognosis is good, with a 10-year survival rate of more than 95%.

50. B (Brooks et al. 1991, 125–126). Transplantation of an individual's own tissue is an autograft and is regularly accepted by the body. An isograft (syngeneic graft) is a transfer of tissue between genetically identical individuals and is usually accepted by the body. A homograft (allograft) is a graft btween genetically different members of the same species, and survival of the transplant is dependent on the matching of the histocompatibility antigens and the use of immunosuppressive drugs. A heterograft (xenograft) is a transfer of tissue between different species and is always rejected. In humans, the major histocompatibility complex is located on the short arm of chromosome 6. Kidneys are the most frequently transplanted organ and have a 5-year survival rate of 95% with a two-haplotype match of related donors, and a 60% rate with cadaver donors. A graft-versus-host reaction may occur in 60% of bone marrow transplants. In this reaction, grafted immunocompetent T cells proliferate in the host and reject host tissue antigens. The reaction may be reduced by eliminating mature T cells from the graft before transplantation (Brooks et al. 1991).

References

Berkow R, Fletcher AJ (eds): The Merck Manual. 15th ed. Rahway, NJ: Merck, 1987.

Brooks GF, et al: Medical Microbiology. 19th ed. Norwalk, CT: Appleton & Lange, 1991.

Dulbecco R, Ginsberg HS: Virology. 2nd ed. Philadelphia: Lippincott, 1988.

Joklik WK, et al. (eds): Zinsser Microbiology. 20th ed. Norwalk, CT: Appleton & Lange, 1992.

Pharmacology

1. The renal clearance of a compound is 100 ml per minute at a steady state of infusion. When the infusion rate is decreased by one half and a new steady state is reached,
   A. the clearance will decrease to 5 ml per minute
   B. the rate of excretion will decrease even if the clearance remains at 100 ml per minute
   C. the volume of distribution will double so that the clearance will remain constant
   D. the clearance would decrease if the compound were being excreted solely by glomerular filtration
   E. None of the above is accurate.

2. The graph below shows the plasma concentration of drug A at various times after intravenous administration of the drug. The drug is known to be distributed in extracellular fluid. The half-life of drug A is
   A. 1 hour
   B. 2 hours
   C. 4 hours
   D. 6 hours
   E. not able to be determined from the information given

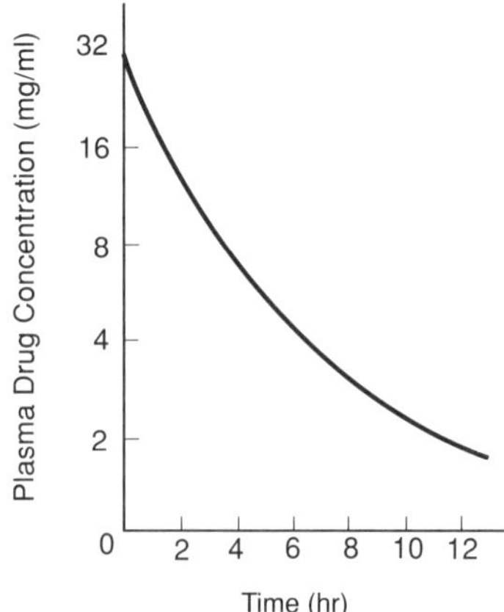

3. A drug that is used therapeutically to produce sleep causes hypotension as an undesirable side effect. Which of the following statements is **not** supported by the data in the graph below?
   A. At a serum concentration of 10 mg/L, 50% of the subjects will be hypotensive.

B. The LD50 of the drug is about 200 mg/L.
C. Every subject falls asleep before becoming hypotensive.
D. These data are presented as quantal dose-response curves.
E. At a serum drug concentration of 1 mg/L, more than 75% of subjects are not asleep.

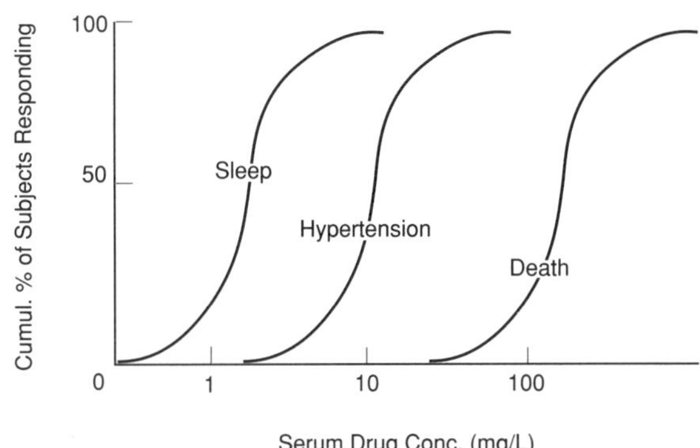

4. Which of the following pharmacokinetic parameters is **least** affected by age?
   A. gastrointestinal absorption
   B. hepatic metabolism
   C. plasma protein binding
   D. renal excretion
   E. tissue distribution

Items 5–8

Match the drug from the lettered list of choices below to the statement with which it is most closely associated. Each choice may be used once, more than once, or not at all.

A. *N*-acetylcysteine
B. pralidoxime
C. dimercaprol (BAL)
D. naloxone
E. amyl nitrite

5. Used as an antidote for both arsenic and inorganic lead poisoning.
6. Used to treat acetaminophen poisoning; acts by increasing liver glutathione levels.
7. Used primarily to treat the nicotinic effects of organophosphates.
8. Used to treat cyanide poisoning; acts by inducing methemoglobinemia.

Items 9–11

Match the drug from the lettered list of choices to the statment with which it is most closely associated. Each lettered choice may be used once, more than once, or not at all.

A. amitriptyline
B. buproprion

C. carbamazepine
D. clozapine
E. desipramine
F. fluoxetine
G. fluphenazine
H. phenelzine
I. pimozide
J. thioridazine

9. Alternative to lithium in the treatment of bipolar diseases.
10. Indicated (in the US) only for the treatment of Tourette's syndrome.
11. Exerts its antidepressant effect primarily by an action on serotonergic systems.

12. After a single oral dose, diazepam has a rapid onset of action and a short duration of action because
    A. it is not converted to active metabolites
    B. it is converted to active metabolites
    C. it is not very highly bound to plasma proteins
    D. of its high lipid solubility
    E. None of these is correct.

13. Many anesthetic agents produce at least some degree of analgesia as well. Which drug in the list below provides **no** analgesic effect?
    A. desflurane
    B. halothane
    C. ketamine
    D. nitrous oxide
    E. thiopental

14. Local anesthetics can produce full nerve blockage by
    A. blocking 10% of the sodium channels
    B. blocking 10% of the potassium channels
    C. blocking 95% of the sodium channels
    D. blocking 95% of the potassium channels
    E. blocking 10% of the calcium channels

15. Which of the following statements is most accurate regarding the minimum anesthetic concentation (MAC)?
    A. MAC is greater for halothane than enflurane (in humans).
    B. MAC is greater for potent as compared to less potent agents.
    C. MAC is smaller for potent as compared to less potent agents.
    D. MAC is lower for N_2O as compared to most other anesthetics (in humans).
    E. MAC is the measure of cardiovascular depression produced by anesthetics.

16. Beta-endorphin–induced analgesia is mediated by the release of which one of the following neurotransmitters?
    A. met-enkephalin
    B. norepinephrine

C. serotonin
D. substance P
E. all of the above

17. The most effective agent in aborting an acute attack of migraine headache is
A. clonidine
B. ergotamine tartrate
C. methysergide
D. propranolol
E. verapamil

18. If the rank order of selectivity of a series of drugs is as follows:

phenylephrine > epinephrine > isoproterenol

then the effect is most likely to be acting through which of the following receptors?
A. $alpha_1$
B. $alpha_2$
C. $beta_1$
D. $beta_2$
E. muscarinic (M_1)

19. the antianginal efficacy of nitroglycerin may be attributed to all of the following effects **except**
A. dilation of collateral blood vessels
B. dilation of large coronary arteries
C. increase in subepicardial blood flow
D. reduction in cardiac work
E. reduction in diastolic wall tension

20. The most important **primary** effect of the cardiac glycosides in the treatment of congestive heart failure is
A. an increase in arterial blood pressure
B. an increase in myocardial contractile force
C. a decrease in heart rate
D. a reduction in cardiac size
E. diuresis

Items 21–23

For each of the diuretic agents listed below, select the mechanism of action that is most appropriate. Each lettered choice may be used once, more than once, or not at all.

A. ethacrynic acid
B. hydrochlorothiazide
C. mercaptomerin
D. spironolactone
E. triamterene

21. Inhibits electrolyte reabsorption in the thick ascending limb of the loop of Henle; increases renal blood flow but does not affect glomerular filtration rate.
22. Inhibits Cl^- reabsorption, especially in the distal portion of the ascending loop of Henle and the early portion of the distal tubule.
23. Inhibits active Na^+ reabsorption and should be used with caution in patients with gout.

24. Which of the following statements is **not correct** regarding the osmotic diuretics?
    A. They are filtered at the glomerulus.
    B. They do not have a marked impact on sodium and chloride ion excretion.
    C. They can be used to reduce cerebrospinal fluid pressure.
    D. They reduce blood volume.
    E. They are poorly reabsorbed due to their molecular size.

25. Which of the following statements regarding clot lysis using streptokinase is **not correct**?
    A. It can cause systemic fibrinogen depletion.
    B. It stimulates the conversion of fibrinogen to fibrin.
    C. It may be ineffective in patients with recent *Strep.* throat infection.
    D. It converts plasminogen to plasmin.
    E. It may produce allergic reactions as a side effect.

26. Which of the following statements about heparin is correct?
    A. It binds to platelet glycoprotein Ib.
    B. It inhibits lipoprotein lipase release.
    C. It is teratogenic.
    D. It promotes conversion of plasminogen to plasmin.
    E. It requries a cofactor, antithrombin III, to be efficacious.

27. Which of the following statements about cholinergics is **not correct**?
    A. Scopolamine HBr is used to treat anterior uveitis in the event of allergic reactions to atropine HBr.
    B. Bethanechol is used to induce miosis for surgery on the anterior region of the eye.
    C. Edrophonium is used in diagnosing myasthenia gravis.
    D. Controlled hypotension is produced by slow IV infusion of trimethaphan during vascular surgery.
    E. Pilocarpine is often used in conjunction with mannitol and acetazolamide in the treatment of angle-closure glaucoma.

28. Which of the following is a stimulus in promoting the production of erythropoietin?
    A. colony-stimulating factor
    B. decompensated renal disease
    C. hypoxia
    D. interleukin-3
    E. thrombocytopenia

Items 29–31

Match each drug in the following list of pharmacologic agents to the statement with which it is most closely associated. Each lettered choice may be used once, more than once, or not at all.

A. betazole
B. serotonin
C. dinoprostone
D. terfenadine
E. ranitidine

29. Used as an alternative to histamine phosphate in tests of gastric function.
30. Approved treatment for patients with gastric esophageal reflux.
31. Effective in relieving seasonal rhinitis, it has no CNS sedating effect.

32. If you were treating a patient for asthmatic bronchospasm, you would prescribe
A. aspirin
B. cromolyn sodium
C. phenylephrine
D. propranolol
E. terbutaline

33. Which of the following statements is **incorrect** regarding indomethacin?
A. It is well tolerated compared to other antiinflammatory agents.
B. It is a more potent antiinflammatory agent than aspirin.
C. It is useful in the treatment of acute gout.
D. It is useful in the treatment of ankylosing spondylitis and osteoarthritis.
E. Side effects include nausea, diarrhea, and headache.

34. Gastric motility is enhanced by which class of drugs?
A. aluminum salts
B. calcium channel blockers
C. cholinomimetics
D. opiates
E. sympathomimetics

35. Gout patients classified as "overproducers" respond
A. better to probenecid than allopurinol
B. minimally to both probenecid and sulfinpyrazone
C. equally well to allopurinol and probenecid
D. minimally to allopurinol and sulfinpyrazone
E. minimally to all of the agents mentioned in this question

36. Antacids, in addition to neutralizing gastric acid secretion, also affect the bowel. Which of the following antacids may produce diarrhea?
A. aluminum hydroxide
B. licorice root
C. magnesium hydroxide

D. sodium bicarbonate
E. Constipation is the side effect, not diarrhea.

37. Of the following agents, which is **not** a standard treatment for hyperlipoproteinemia?
A. lovastatin
B. nystatin
C. nicotinic acid
D. neomycin
E. probucol

38. Which of the following **is not** a physiologic or pharmacologic effect of insulin?
A. inhibition of gluconeogenesis
B. stimulation of glycogen synthesis
C. stimulation of lipid synthesis
D. stimulation of lipolysis
E. stimulation of protein synthesis

39. Which is the drug of choice for the medical management of hyperprolactinemia?
A. bromocriptine
B. cyproheptadine
C. clomiphene
D. somatostatin
E. none of the above

40. A ligand for a receptor is identified and found to have a K_D of 1 nm and an alpha of 0. This evidence is compatible with the ligand being
A. an agonist
B. a partial agonist
C. a partial antagonist
D. an antagonist
E. none of the above

41. Which of the following **is not** a principle of combination therapy of neoplastic diseases?
A. All drugs in the combination should be effective as single agents unless used for "rescue."
B. Toxicities of the drugs used should be the same.
C. All drugs should be used at their optimal dose and schedule.
D. Drugs in a combination regimen should have different mechanisms of action to avoid development of resistance.
E. All of these are correct principles of combination chemotherapy.

42. Identify the **incorrectly** matched pair in the following list.

A. cisplatin	Used for genitourinary cancer and highly nephrotoxic.
B. methotrexate	Incorporated into DNA; causes myelosuppression.

C. 5-fluorouracil	Metabolite covalently binds to thymidylate synthetase.
D. vincristine	Used in childhood leukemia; is neurotoxic.
E. tamoxifen	A competitive inhibitor of estrogen binding; used in estrogen receptor-positive breast cancer.

43. All of the following are correct statements regarding antihypertensive agents **except**
   A. sudden withdrawal of metoprolol is extremely dangerous
   B. hydralazine promotes a baroreflex increase in heart rate and contractility
   C. chlorothiazide can lead to hypokalemia, hyperuricemia, hyperlipoproteinemia, and hyperglycemia
   D. diltiazem is the drug of choice in hypertensives with congestive heart failure
   E. captopril is well tolerated, but may cause a chronic cough and rise in serum potassium

44. Which of the following groups of cancer chemotherapeutic agents inhibit purine ring biosynthesis?
   A. 6-mercaptopurine, thioguanine, and methotrexate
   B. colchicine, thioguanine, and methotrexate
   C. mitomycin and cisplatin
   D. hydroxyurea and cytarabine
   E. asparaginase and 5-fluorouracil

45. The hospital laboratory has just informed you that an India ink stain of the spinal fluid from one of your patients is positive for *Cryptococcus neoformans*. Which of the following would be an appropriate first-choice therapy?
   A. oral amphotericin combined with intravenous miconazole
   B. oral amphotericin alone
   C. intravenous amphotericin combined with intravenous ketoconazole
   D. all of the above
   E. none of the above

46. You are seeing a patient who has just been diagnosed with malaria. The drug of first choice in treating this patient is
   A. amphotericin B
   B. chloroquine
   C. ivermectin
   D. praziquantel
   E. tetracycline

47. Antiviral drugs that inhibit nucleic acid synthesis include
   A. amantadine and vidarabine
   B. amantadine and rimantadine
   C. methisazone, rifampin, and idoxuridine
   D. AZT, methisazone, and 2',3'-dideoxycytidine
   E. interferon, vidarabine, and acyclovir

48. Which of the following antibiotics **does not** act via inhibition of bacterial cell wall synthesis?
    A. vancomycin
    B. penicillin G
    C. bacitracin
    D. cephalosporins
    E. quinolones

49. It is well known that long-term treatment of hypertension with propranolol produces an increase in the number of beta-adrenergic receptors in the heart. This is an example of
    A. desensitization
    B. enhanced affinity
    C. tachyphylaxis
    D. receptor upregulation
    E. synergism

50. A primary action of folic acid is to
    A. transport vitamin B_{12} to reactive sites
    B. protect against oxidation of iron compounds
    C. enhance production of erythropoietin
    D. provide methyl groups to convert uridylic to thymidylic acid
    E. protect against proliferation of malignant cells

51. Serum theophylline levels tend to become increased in which of the following groups?
    A. patients treated with carbamazepine
    B. smokers
    C. patients receiving phenobarbital
    D. patients receiving erythromycin
    E. patients receiving phenytoin (dilantin)

52. Which of the following anesthetic combinations would produce the **least** cardiac depressant effect?
    A. enflurane plus nitrous oxide
    B. enflurane plus propofol
    C. nitrous oxide plus halothane
    D. ketamine plus nitrous oxide
    E. halothane plus thiopental

Explanations for Pharmacology Items

1. B

2. C (Gilman et al. 1990, 24–26). The half-life of a drug is the time required for the plasma concentration of the compound to decline by 50% ($t_{1/2}$). This semilogarithmic graph illustrates a two-compartment model of IV drug administration. The time required for a 50% reduction of the drug during the elimination phase of the curve ($t_{1/2}B$) is 4 hours (at 8

hours, plasma concentration is 4 µ/ml; at 12 hours, plasma concentration is 2µg/ml).

3. C

4. A

5. C

6. A (Gilman et al. 1990, 658). Acetaminophen is metabolized in the liver primarily by conjugation with glucuronic acid (60%), sulfuric acid (35%), or cysteine (3%), although a small proportion of the drug undergoes cytochrome P_{450}-mediated i-hydroxylation to form a highly reactive n-acetyl-benzoquinoneimine. This metabolite reacts with sulfhydryl groups in glutathione, and with the sulfhydryl group of hepatic proteins upon depletion of glutathione. n-Acetylcysteine replenishes hepatic stores of glutathione, thereby reducing the hepatotoxicity induced by n-acetyl-benzoquinoneimine on overdosing of acetaminophen.

7. B (Gilman et al. 1990, 132–142). Organophosphates inhibit acetylcholinesterase by binding to the active site of the enzyme, thereby preventing the termination of acetylcholine activity at cholinergic nerve endings. Parlidoxime (2-PAM) reactivates the enzyme via nucleophilic attack on the phosphorus of organophosphates, freeing the active site to bind acetylcholine.

8. E

9. C

10. I

11. F (Gilman et al. 1990, 405–414). Fluoxetine (Prozac) is a serotonin uptake inhibitor used to treat depression. It has minimal binding affinity for cholinergic, histaminergic, and alpha-adrenergic receptors, which are sources of adverse side effects associated with other antidepressants.

12. D

13. E

14. C (Gilman et al. 1990, 311–319). Both amide- and ester-linked local anesthetics block the propagation of neuronal action potentials in a circumscribed area of the body. The main site of drug action is voltage-sensitive sodium channels, where local anesthetics bind to block sodium conductance, thus depressing membrane depolarization. In addition to sodium channels, local anesthetics can bind to other membrane-bound proteins, such as potassium channels, but this is not the major site of action at clinically relevant doses.

15. C

16. A

17. B (Gilman et al. 1990, 945–947). Ergotamine is the drug of choice for symptomatic relief of acute migraine attack, and is very efficacious in most cases. Propranolol is the preferred drug for prophylaxis of migraine headaches, although methysergide, calcium channel blockers (verapamil), and tricyclic antidepressants are also effective prophylactic agents.

18. A (Gilman et al. 1990, 106–110). Phenylephrine is a specific, postsynaptic $alpha_1$ agonist. Epinephrine acts at both beta and alpha receptors, displaying a higher affinity for beta receptors. Thus, epinephrine is less selective than phenylephrine for $alpha_1$ receptors. Isoproterenol is a potent, nonselective beta agonist, and has far less affinity for alpha receptors than do phenylephrine and epinephrine.

19. C

20. B (Gilman et al. 1990, 825–827). Increased myocardial contractility is the primary beneficial effect of cardiac glycosides in the treatment of congestive heart failure. As a result of direct positive inotropic action, cardiac glycosides secondarily increase cardiac output, decrease heart size and heart rate, and decrease venous and capillary pressures. Furthermore, the improved hemodynamic state leads to a reduction in neural and humoral vasoconstrictor mechanisms, resulting in a decrease in systemic vascular resistance and enhanced renal blood flow.

21. A

22. B

23. E

24. D

25. B (Gilman et al. 1990, 1323). Streptokinase noncovalently complexes with plasminogen to allow cleavage of arginine 560, converting plasminogen to plasmin. Plasmin lacks fibrin specificity, inducing a systemic lytic state, causing fibrinogenolysis. Prior streptococcal infections produce antibodies capable of inactivating streptokinase. Adverse side effects of streptokinase include allergic reactions, anaphylaxis, and fever. Thrombin, not streptokinase, converts fibrinogen to fibrin.

26. E

27. B (Gilman et al. 1990, 122–127, 143–145, 162, 181–184). Bethanechol is a muscarinic agonist that selectively acts in the smooth muscle of the GI and urinary tracts. It is given subcutaneously to treat postpartum urinary retention and opiate-induced bowel stasis. Acetylcholine and carbachol are commonly used to induce miosis during eye surgery.

28. C (Gilman et al. 1990, 1279–1282). Erythropoietin is a growth factor produced by the kidney that is responsible for erythropoiesis. Renal blood oxygen sensors signal rapid secretion of erythropoietin during periods of hypoxia. While erythropoietin is not the only growth factor associated with red cell production, lack of this protein causes severe anemia.

29. A

30. E (Gilman et al. 1990, 899–902). Ranitidine (Zantac) is an H_2 antagonist that inhibits gastric acid secretion elicited by histamine, gastrin, and, to a lesser extent, muscarinic agonists. Therapeutic uses of ranitidine include treatment of duodenal and gastric ulcers, Zollinger-Ellison syndrome, and reflux esophagitis.

31. D (Gilman et al. 1990, 582–587). H_1 antagonists are effective drugs for the relief of allergy symptoms such as rhinitis, urticaria, and conjunctivitis. Terfenadine (Seldane), a new-generation drug, is excluded from the brain, preventing the CNS side effects of restlessness and sedation associated with older H_1 antagonists.

32. E

33. A (Gilman et al. 1990, 659–661). Indomethacin is an older nonsteriodal antiinflammatory agent originally produced for the treatment of rheumatoid arthritis. It is more potent than aspirin in relieving the symptoms of ankylosing spondylitis and osteoarthritis and is also an effective treatment of acute gout. A large percentage of patients experience effects from indomethacin therapy (anorexia, nausea, diarrhea, and severe frontal headache). Because it is not as well tolerated as other antiinflammatory agents, indomethacin is not routinely used for its analgesic or antipyretic properties.

34. C

35. B (Gilman et al. 1990, 676–679). Uricosuric agents such as probenecid and sulfinpyrazone inhibit the reabsorption of urate via competition for the brush-border transporter of the kidney. Overproduction of uric acid promotes the formation of xanthine oxidase, thereby decreasing uric acid synthesis. Since "overproducers" synthesize uric acid faster than urocosurics can excrete the compound, allopurinol is the drug of choice for treating gout in patients with hyperuricemia, as well as those with impaired renal function.

36. C (Gilman et al. 1990, 904–909). In addition to neutralizing acid, magnesium hydroxide is also an osmotic purgative agent, causing diarrhea by drawing water into the bowel and stimulating cholecystokinin release. Sodium bicarbonate has little effect on bowel motility; aluminum hydroxide causes constipation in a dose-dependent manner. Licorice root has been used as an antacid, but its effect is probably due to its demulcent effect, soothing irritated mucous tissues within the GI tract.

37. B

38. D (Gilman et al. 1990, 1468–1475). Insulin inhibits hepatic glucose synthesis (gluconeogenesis) and stimulates uptake and metabolism of glucose by muscle and adipose tissue, thereby reducing blood glucose levels. Insulin promotes storage of glucose in the liver (glycogen synthesis), triglyceride formation (lipid synthesis), and the storage of amino acids in muscle (protein synthesis). Insulin inhibits the breakdown of triglycerides (lipolysis) and the conversion of amino acids to glucose (gluconeogenesis).

39. A

40. D

41. B (Gilman et al. 1990, 1202–1257; Bennett 1992, 1499–1507). Employing drugs with differing levels of toxicity alows the administration of maximal doses of each compound during combination therapy. Answers A, C, and D are principles of combination therapy that should be followed.

42. B

43. D

44. A

45. E (Gilman et al. 1990, 1165–1172). Amphotericin B (Fungizone) increases fungal membrane permeability and is effective for treating systemic fungal infections. It synergizes with flucytosine to improve the sensitivity of *Cryptococcus neoformans* to antifungal therapy. Poor GI absorption necessitates IV administration of amphotericin B. Ketoconazole is given orally, and both ketoconazole and miconazole do not penetrate the CSF. Therefore, the answer is "none of the above."

46. B

47. E (Gilman et al. 1990, 1182–1196). Interferons have multiple mechanisms of action, such as inhibiting viral penetration of cells, inhibiting the synthesis or methylation of mRNA, preventing the translation of viral proteins, or inhibiting the assembly and release of viruses. Acyclovir and vidarabine inhibit viral DNA polymerase, thereby, preventing DNA synthesis. Azidothymidine (AZT, Retrovir) inhibits viral reverse transcriptase, blocking DNA synthesis. Idoxuridine is incorporated into DNA, making the nucleic acid more susceptible to strand breaks. This causes RNA transcription errors and the production of faulty viral proteins. Rimantadine and amantadine prevent assembly of influenza A virus, but have no effect on nucleic acid synthesis. Methisazone, a prophylactic agent for smallpox, prevents proper viral mRNA translation, but it has little clinical use today. Rifampin and 2', 3'-dideoxycytidine are not commonly used as antiviral agents.

48. E

49. D

50. D (Gilman et al. 1990, 1302–1306). Folic acid is an essential vitamin that donates methyl groups for the synthesis of DNA precursors. Leucovorin (folinic acid) circumvents dihydrofolate reductase inhibition by promoting the conversion of uridylic acid to thymidate, thereby "rescuing" normal cells from methotrexate toxicity. The hematopoietic system is sensitive to folate deficiency, as the rapid turnover of blood cells requires active DNA synthesis. Folate is not responsible for erythropoietin production or cyanocobalamin transport.

51. D (Gilman et al. 1990, 627). Methylxanthines such as theophylline are metabolized in the liver via demethylation, oxidation, and hydroxylation. Agents known to block hepatic metabolism of theophylline (cimetidine, verapamil, and erythromycin) reduce the clearance of the methylxanthine, thereby increasing its serum concentration. Smoking and barbiturates (Dilantin and phenobarbital) increase the clearance of theophylline, which reduces its serum levels. Carbamazepine is conjugated and hydroxylated in the liver, and, like theophylline, has increased clearance in the presence of phenobarbital and Dilantin.

52. D

References

Bennett DR (ed): AMA Drug Evaluations. 5th ed. Chicago: American Medical Association, 1992.

Gilman AG, et al. (eds): The Pharmacological Basis of Therapeutics. 8th ed. New York: Pergamon, 1990.

Index